COLOR ATLAS
OF
CLINICAL
EMBRYOLOGY

COLOR ATLAS OF CLINICAL EMBRYOLOGY

KEITH L. MOORE, B.A., M.Sc., Ph.D., F.I.A.C., F.R.S.M.

Professor of Anatomy and Cell Biology
Faculty of Medicine, University of Toronto
Toronto, Ontario, Canada

Visiting Professor of Clinical Anatomy
Department of Anatomy, Faculty of Medicine
University of Manitoba
Winnipeg, Manitoba, Canada

T.V.N. PERSAUD, M.D., Ph.D., D.Sc., F.R.C. Path. (Lond.)

Professor and Former Head, Department of Anatomy
Professor of Pediatrics and Child Health
Associate Professor of Obstetrics, Gynecology and
    Reproductive Sciences
University of Manitoba, Faculties of Medicine and Dentistry

Consultant in Pathology and Clinical Genetics
Health Sciences Centre
Winnipeg, Manitoba, Canada

KOHEI SHIOTA, M.D., D.Med.Sc.

Professor and Chairman
Department of Anatomy and Developmental Biology
Director of Congenital Anomaly Research Center
Faculty of Medicine
Kyoto University
Kyoto, Japan

W. B. SAUNDERS COMPANY
A Division of Harcourt Brace & Company

Philadelphia, London, Toronto, Montreal, Sydney, Tokyo

W. B. SAUNDERS COMPANY
A Division of Harcourt Brace & Company

The Curtis Center
Independence Square West
Philadelphia, PA 19106

Library of Congress Cataloging-in-Publication Data

Moore, Keith L.
    Color atlas of clinical embryology / Keith L. Moore, T.V.N. Persaud, Kohei Shiota.
       p.   cm.
    Includes bibliographical references and index.
    ISBN 0-7216-4663-8
    1. Embryology. Human--Atlases. I. Persaud, T. V. N. II. Shiota, Kohei. III. Title.
    [DNLM: 1. Fetal Development--atlases. 2. Abnormalities--atlases. QS 617
M822e 1994]
QM602.M66 1994
611'.013'0222--dc20
DNLM/DLC   93-26435

COLOR ATLAS OF CLINICAL EMBRYOLOGY   ISBN 0-7216-4663-8

Printed in the United States of America.

Last digit is the print number: 9   8   7   6   5   4   3   2   1

Dedicated to a greater understanding of life
and to
our wives and children

Illustrations

Sari O'Sullivan, B.F.A., B.Sc., AAM
Valda Glennie, B.A., B.Sc., AAM
Heinz Loth, B.Sc., AAM
David Mazierski, B.Sc., AAM
Glenn Reid, B.Sc., AAM

Photographs

Paul Schwartz, B.A.
Stephen Epstein
Toshiaki Nagai

Keyboarding

Marion Moore, B.A.

Microdissection

Chigako Uwabe, B.Sc.

PREFACE

The reproductive revolution in the last decade has resulted in rapid advances in our understanding of human embryology and in techniques for assessing the status of developing humans. Human embryos and fetuses have become medicine's newest patients.

*The aim of this color atlas is to give a well-illustrated **overview of life before birth**.* The color photographs, drawings, electron micrographs, sonograms, MRIs, and pen and ink sketches give an appreciation of embryos and fetuses at various stages of development and indicate periods when the formation of the tissues and organs may be affected by teratogenic agents (e.g., drugs, viruses, and radiation). Some photographs have been color-enhanced to show the natural appearance of the embryos, fetuses, and their associated membranes.

*The atlas provides a **visual summary of human development*** and an outline of the most important developmental concepts. It should be useful to all health care professionals, but it will likely be most helpful to clinical geneticists, dysmorphologists, embryologists, embryopathologists, maternity nurses, medical students, medicolegal experts, obstetricians, pediatricians, and perinatalogists. The introductory statements at the beginning of each chapter and the legends to the illustrations provide an overview of the main stages and crucial events of life before birth. The principal systems involved in congenital anomalies are also illustrated and photomicrographs of various tissues and organs are described. Selected serial sections of embryos during the period when most defects originate are also included.

We have been most fortunate in the expert assistance we have received from several medical photographers: Paul Schwartz and Stephen Epstein in Creative Communications, Instructional Media Services, Faculty of Medicine, University of Toronto, and Toshiaki Nagai in the Department of Anatomy, Faculty of Medicine, Kyoto University, Kyoto, Japan. Our principal medical illustrators were Sari O'Sullivan, David Mazierski, and Valda Glennie. Without their expert skill and desire to achieve excellence in their art, the quality of this atlas could not have been attained. We are also most grateful to Ms. Chigako Uwabe of the Congenital Anomaly Research Center, Faculty of Medicine, Kyoto University. She examined most of the embryos in the collection and did the microdissections of the embryos illustrated in this atlas. We are very grateful to Marion Moore, who typed the manuscript, proofread it, and helped with the design of the Atlas.

We acknowledge with much pleasure our gratitude to Professor Hideo Nishimura and his colleagues in Kyoto University, who developed the Congenital Anomaly Research Center. We are also grateful to Professor Kasumasa Hoshino, his successor as Professor and Chairman of Anatomy and Director of the Congenital Anomaly Research Center for permitting us to prepare photographs of many of the specimens for use in this atlas. The senior author is also grateful to him for the honor of spending several weeks studying the embryos in the world-renowned Kyoto collection. Dr. Albert E. Chudley, Head of Genetics and Metabolism and Professor of Pediatrics and Child Health and Professor of Human Genetics in the Faculty of Medicine, University of Manitoba, and Dr. Dagmar K. Kalousek, Program Head, Cytogenetics/Embryopathology Laboratory and Professor of Pathology in the University of British Columbia, Vancouver, B.C., Canada, provided many of the photographs of embryos, fetuses, and neonates with congenital anomalies. Barbara Paradice in Dr. Kalousek's laboratory was also most helpful. We are grateful to Dr. Raymond F. Gasser, Professor of Anatomy at Louisiana State University, Medical Center, New Orleans, Louisiana, for help with the presentation of the serial sections of human embryos. His expertise in this area is widely recognized. We are also grateful to others who kindly provided illustrations for the atlas. Their contributions are acknowledged in the legends to the figures.

KEITH L. MOORE

T.V.N. PERSAUD

KOHEI SHIOTA

CONTENTS

1
THE FIRST TWO WEEKS OF HUMAN DEVELOPMENT

Human development begins at **fertilization** (conception) when an oocyte (ovum) from a woman is fertilized by a sperm (spermatozoon) from a man. Union of these *gametes* (germ cells) during fertilization produces a **zygote** or fertilized ovum (Fig. 1–1), which is the primordium or *beginning of a new human being.* Formation of the zygote normally occurs in the ampulla of the uterine tube (fallopian tube), the longest and widest part of the tube (Fig. 1–3). *In vitro fertilization* (IVF) of an oocyte in a Petri dish (Fig. 1–2) provides the opportunity to alleviate infertility resulting from blocked uterine tubes (Moore and Persaud, 1993).

Fertilization initiates embryonic development by stimulating the zygote to undergo a series of mitotic cell divisions called **cleavage.** First, the zygote divides into two cells called *blastomeres* (Figs. 1–1 to 1–3). These primordial cells soon divide to form four blastomeres, eight blastomeres, and so on. Cleavage normally occurs as the zygote passes along the uterine tube toward the uterus (Fig. 1–3). During cleavage the blastomeres change their shape and size and tightly align themselves against each other to form a compact ball of blastomeres known as a morula (L. *morus,* mulberry). The **morula,** a cluster of 12 to 16 blastomeres, *forms about three days after fertilization,* just before entering the uterus (Figs. 1–1 and 1–3). Shortly after *the morula enters the uterus,* fluid-filled spaces appear between its central blastomeres. Soon the cells are separated into two parts: (1) a thin outer cell layer called the *trophoblast,* which forms the fetal part of the placenta, and (2) a group of centrally located blastomeres which forms the **inner cell mass** or *embryoblast,* the primordium of the embryo. The conceptus is now known as a blastocyst (Figs. 1–1 and 1–3).

The **blastocyst** floats freely in the uterine cavity for about two days. While floating in the uterus, the blastocyst derives its nourishment from the secretions of the uterine glands (Figs. 1–4 and 1–5). About six days after fertilization (day 20 of a 28-day menstrual cycle),[1] *the blastocyst attaches to the endometrial epithelium* (Figs. 1–1 and 1–3). As this occurs, **the trophoblast proliferates** to form two layers: (1) an inner *cytotrophoblast* (cellular trophoblast) and (2) an outer *syncytiotrophoblast* (syncytial trophoblast). Fingerlike processes of the syncytiotrophoblast extend through the endometrial epithelium by secreting substances that erode the endometrial tissues. By the end of the first week, the blastocyst is superficially implanted in the endometrium (Figs. 1–1 and 1–3), and derives its nourishment and oxygen from the maternal endometrial tissues.

At eight to nine days, the **amniotic cavity** appears as a space between the cytotrophoblast and embryoblast (Fig. 1–5). *Amnioblasts* derived from the cytotrophoblast soon line the amniotic cavity and form the **amnion.** As the amniotic sac forms, the *yolk sac* develops and spaces called *lacunae* form in the syncytiotrophoblast.

---

[1]This atlas uses the estimated date of fertilization as the beginning of pregnancy. To obtain *gestational age* (calculated from the last normal menstrual period [Fig. 1–1]), add 14 days to the estimated *fertilization age.*

HUMAN PRENATAL DEVELOPMENT
The First Two Weeks

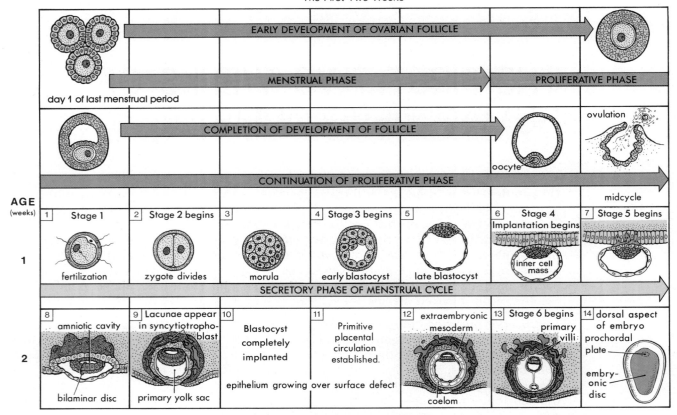

Figure 1–1. Gestational age is calculated from day 1 of the last normal menstrual period (LNMP); however, the embryo does not begin to develop until fertilization of the oocyte occurs about 14 days later. Development of an ovarian follicle and ovulation of the oocyte occur during the first two weeks of the menstrual cycle. Stage 1 of development begins when the oocyte (ovum) is fertilized to form a zygote, about 14 days after LNMP. Cleavage of the zygote occurs during stage 2. The morula enters the uterus on day 3 and the blastocyst forms during stage 3. During stages 4 and 5 the blastocyst attaches to and implants in the endometrium. Stage 6 occurs at the end of the second week when the bilaminar embryonic disc forms and primary chorionic villi appear. (Modified from Moore, KL and Persaud, TVN: *The Developing Human,* ed 5. Philadelphia, WB Saunders, 1993.)

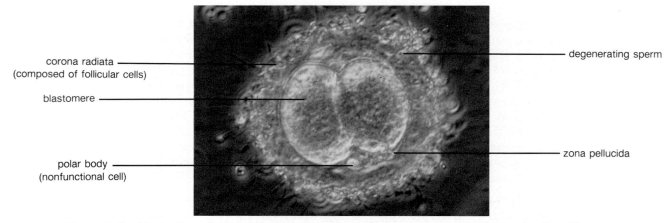

Figure 1–2. Illustration of a two-cell cleaved zygote at Carnegie stage 2, developing in vitro. Observe that it is surrounded by many sperms. Each blastomere has the potential to develop into an embryo. The polar body is a nonfunctional cell. The dividing zygote is observed until the four-to-eight-cell stage and is then placed in the uterus. To increase the chances of pregnancy, three or four cleaved zygotes are inserted into the uterine tube or uterine cavity. (Courtesy of Dr. Maria T. Zenzes and Dr. Peng Wang, In Vitro Fertilization Program, Toronto Hospital, Toronto, Ontario, Canada.)

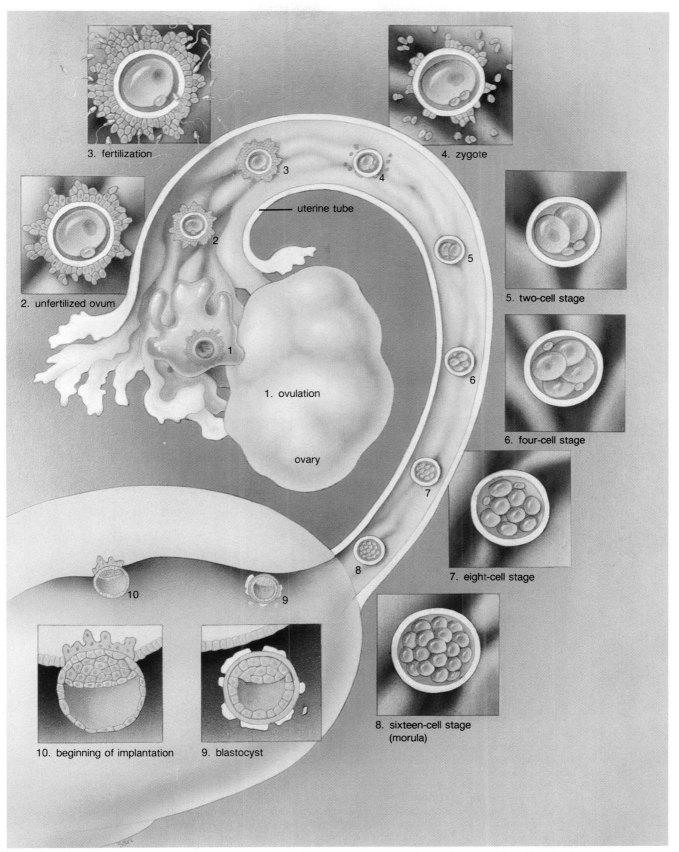

Figure 1–3. Illustration of the first week of human development, showing ovulation, fertilization, and cleavage of the zygote. Observe that the first two stages of development occur in the uterine tube. The morula enters the uterus on day 3 and the blastocyst forms on day 4, stage 3 of development (Fig. 1–1). After floating in the uterus for about two days, the blastocyst begins to implant in the endometrium of the uterus.

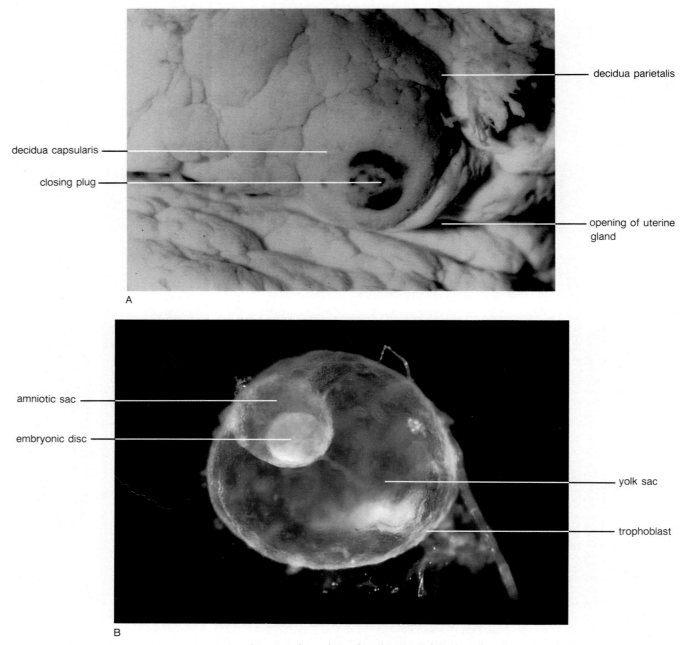

Figure 1–4. *A,* Photograph showing a surface view of an implantation site of a human conceptus at an estimated fertilization age of 14 days. The implanted blastocyst produces a swelling of the endometrium (decidua capsularis) that bulges into the uterine cavity (see Fig. 4–1). The closing plug forms where the blastocyst entered the endometrium. (From Nishimura H (ed): *Atlas of Human Prenatal Histology.* Tokyo, Igaku-Shoin, 1983). *B,* Photograph of a blastocyst during Carnegie stage 6 of development, about 14 days. (From Nishimura et al: *Prenatal Development of the Human with Special Reference to Craniofacial Structures: An Atlas.* US Department of Health, Education and Welfare, NIH, Bethesda, 1977.)

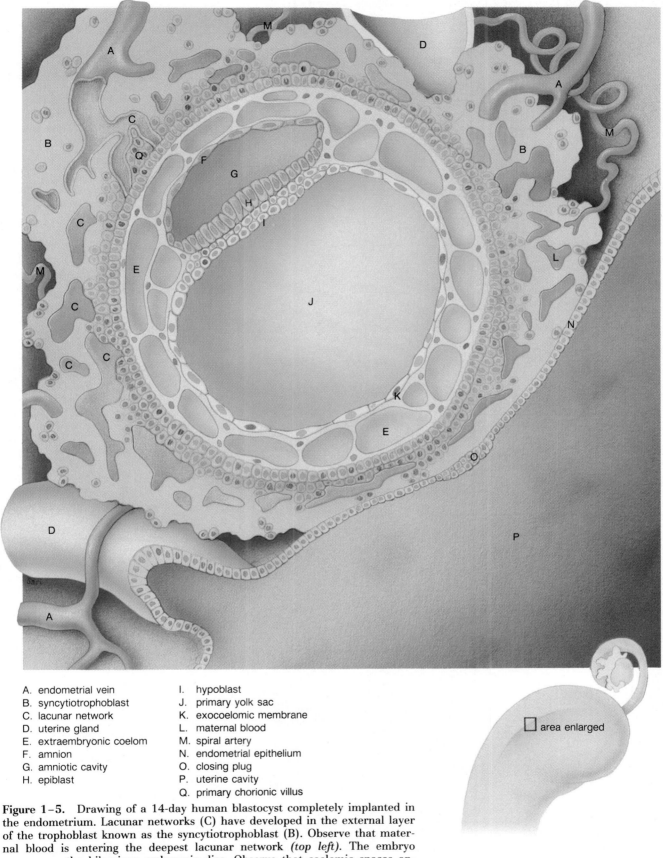

A. endometrial vein
B. syncytiotrophoblast
C. lacunar network
D. uterine gland
E. extraembryonic coelom
F. amnion
G. amniotic cavity
H. epiblast

I. hypoblast
J. primary yolk sac
K. exocoelomic membrane
L. maternal blood
M. spiral artery
N. endometrial epithelium
O. closing plug
P. uterine cavity
Q. primary chorionic villus

☐ area enlarged

Figure 1–5. Drawing of a 14-day human blastocyst completely implanted in the endometrium. Lacunar networks (C) have developed in the external layer of the trophoblast known as the syncytiotrophoblast (B). Observe that maternal blood is entering the deepest lacunar network *(top left)*. The embryo appears as the bilaminar embryonic disc. Observe that coelomic spaces appear in the extraembryonic mesoderm (E). These spaces will fuse to form the extraembryonic coelom (primordium of the chorionic cavity.)

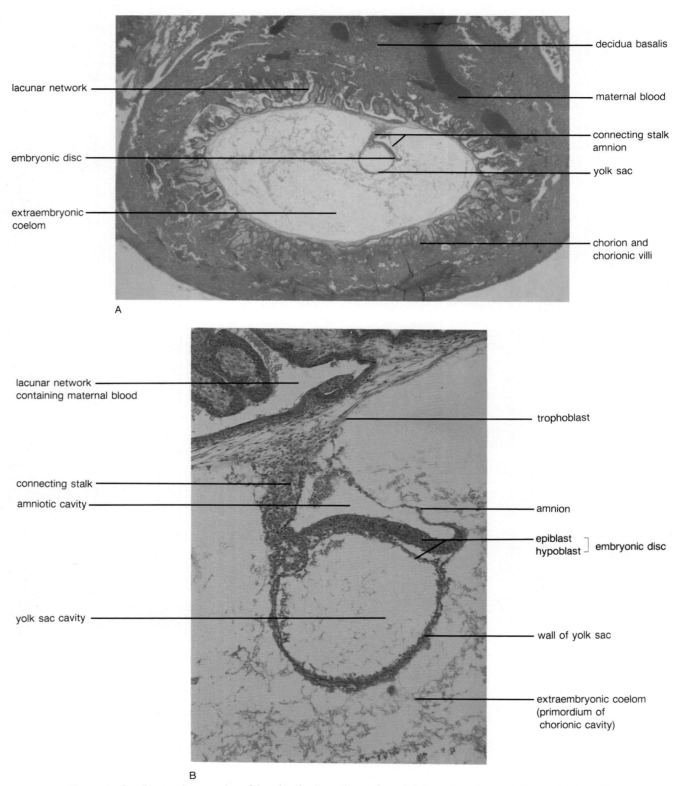

Figure 1–6. Photomicrographs of longitudinal sections of an implanted embryo at Carnegie stage 6, about 14 days. Note the large size of the extraembryonic coelom. *A,* Low-power view (×18). *B,* High-power view (×95). The embryo is represented by the bilaminar embryonic disc composed of epiblast and hypoblast (see also Fig. 1–5). (From Nishimura H (ed): *Atlas of Human Prenatal Histology.* Tokyo, Igaku-Shoin, 1983.)

Fusion of lacunae forms **lacunar networks** that contain maternal blood. Flow of blood through the lacunar networks establishes a primitive *uteroplacental circulation.*

Implantation of the blastocyst is completed by the end of the second week (Figs. 1–4 and 1–5). As this process takes place, changes occur in the embryoblast that produce a **bilaminar embryonic disc,** composed of two layers, *epiblast* and *hypoblast* (Fig. 1–6). As the blastocyst implants in the endometrium, the syncytiotrophoblast produces *human chorionic gonadotropin* (hCG), which enters the maternal blood. This hormone maintains the endometrium and forms the basis for pregnancy testing.

Ectopic pregnancies occur when blastocysts implant outside the uterus, most often in the uterine tube. There are several causes of ectopic pregnancy, but *abnormal sites of implantation* are often related to factors that delay or prevent transportation of the zygote to the uterus. **Spontaneous abortions** are common during the first two weeks due to abnormalities of the blastocysts and problems associated with their implantation. The early *spontaneous abortion rate* is thought to be about 45 per cent.

Throughout this Atlas, references are made to the developmental stages of embryonic development. These numerical stages are based on the **Carnegie Classification System** proposed by O'Rahilly and Müller (1987), which is outlined in Table 5–1 and described in Chapter 5. The Carnegie Collection of embryos is in the Human Developmental Anatomy Center in the National Museum of Health and Medicine, Armed Forces Institute of Pathology, Washington D.C.

2

THE THIRD TO EIGHTH WEEKS OF HUMAN DEVELOPMENT

These six weeks constitute the **embryonic period.** The primordia or beginnings of all major external and internal structures are established during this period. By the end of the eighth week, all main organ systems have begun to develop but the function of most of them is minimal. As the organs form, the shape of the embryo changes so that by 56 days it has a distinctly human appearance.

THE THIRD WEEK

The third week is the beginning of the embryonic period. Rapid development of the embryo from the embryonic disc formed during the second week is characterized by the formation of the primitive streak, notochord, and three **germ layers** from which all tissues and organs develop (Fig. 2–1). The *beginning of morphogenesis* (development of body form) is the most significant event occurring during the third week. Gastrulation, the process that establishes the three germ layers (ectoderm, mesoderm, and endoderm), begins with formation of the **primitive streak** in the epiblast (Figs. 2–1 to 2–3 and 2–6). At 15 days the disclike embryo is oval to round. The primitive streak has a narrow *primitive groove* with slightly bulging folds on each side. Shortly after the primitive streak appears, cells leave its deep surface and form a loose network of embryonic connective tissue called *mesenchyme* (Fig. 2–2B). Some mesenchymal cells form the mesoderm, which the primitive streak actively produces for about two weeks. Normally the streak diminishes in size and becomes an insignificant structure in the future sacrococcygeal region of the embryo. Remnants of the primitive streak may persist and give rise to a tumor known as a *sacrococcygeal teratoma* (Fig. 2–4).

The next structure to appear during the third week is the **notochordal process** (Fig. 2–2C). It is formed by cells derived from the primitive node of the primitive streak. This process grows toward the *prochordal plate* that indicates where the mouth will develop. By the end of the third week the tubelike notochordal process (Fig. 2–2F) has transformed into the **notochord** (Figs. 2–3D and 2–6D). This cellular rod defines the primitive axis of the embryo and gives it some rigidity. It also indicates the future site of the vertebral column (see Chapter 12).

Neurulation is a major event that begins at the end of the third week. It involves formation of the *neural plate, neural folds, neural crest,* and *neural tube* (Figs. 2–3B and 2–5). As these structures form, the intraembryonic mesoderm proliferates to form columns of *paraxial mesoderm.* Each column is continuous laterally with the *intermediate mesoderm* (Fig. 2–6B), which gradually thins laterally into a layer of *lateral mesoderm.* By the end of the third week the cranial ends of the paraxial columns of mesoderm have begun to divide into two to three pairs of cuboidal bodies called **somites** (Figs. 2–5 and 2–6). The somites give rise to most of the axial

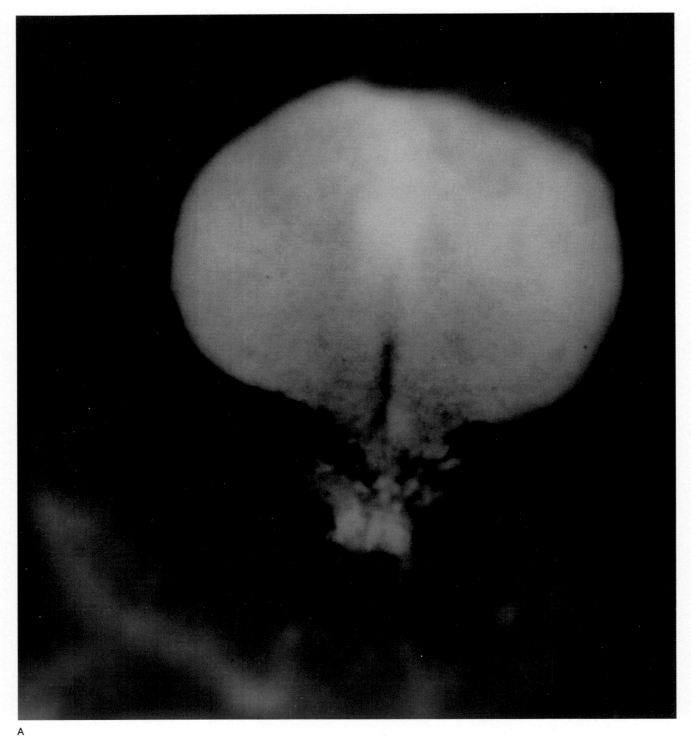

A

Figure 2-1. *A,* Dorsal view of a presomite embryo at Carnegie stage 7, about 16 days. *B,* Diagram indicating the structures shown in *A.* The primitive streak extends caudally from the primitive node (knot) as a zone of ectodermal proliferation in the embryonic disc, the caudal part of which is disrupted. A shallow sulcus, called the primitive groove, is visible, especially in the caudal part of the streak. (From Nishimura, H. and Tanimura, T.: Clinical Aspects of the Teratogenicity of Drugs. Excerpta Medica/American Elsevier, 1976.)

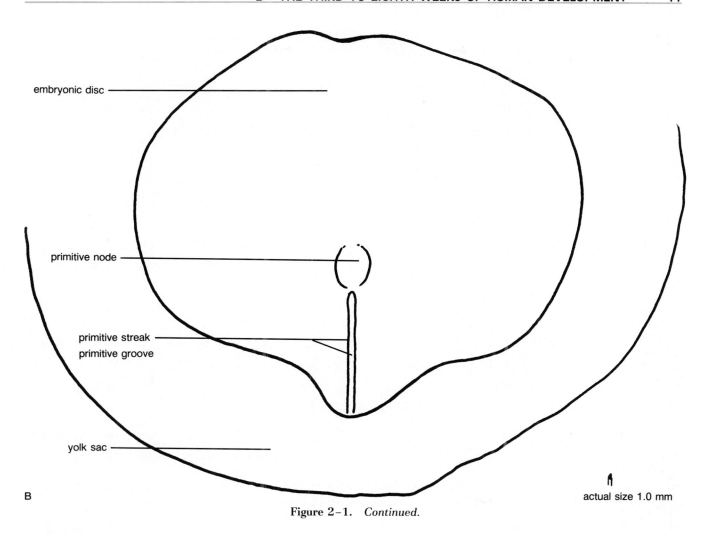

embryonic disc

primitive node

primitive streak
primitive groove

yolk sac

B

actual size 1.0 mm

Figure 2–1. *Continued.*

skeleton. The **intraembryonic coelom** also appears between the layers of lateral mesoderm (Fig. 2–6*D*), which is the primordium of the body cavities (pericardial, pleural, and peritoneal cavities).

Early development of the cardiovascular system also occurs during the third week. The **primordial heart and great vessels** develop from mesenchymal cells in the *cardiogenic area,* located cranial to the prochordal plate (Figs. 2–2 and 2–3). Paired endothelial heart tubes develop and fuse to form a primitive heart tube which is joined to vessels in the embryo, connecting stalk, chorion, and yolk sac (see Chapter 11). *At the end of the third week, the heart begins to beat* and blood begins to circulate through the primitive cardiovascular system.

Chorionic villi, which started to develop at the end of the second week, differentiate into secondary and, later, tertiary villi (primordia of stem villi), which contain *arteriocapillary networks* (see Chapter 4). Oxygen and nutrients now pass from the maternal blood to the fetal blood and carbon dioxide and waste products pass in the opposite direction.

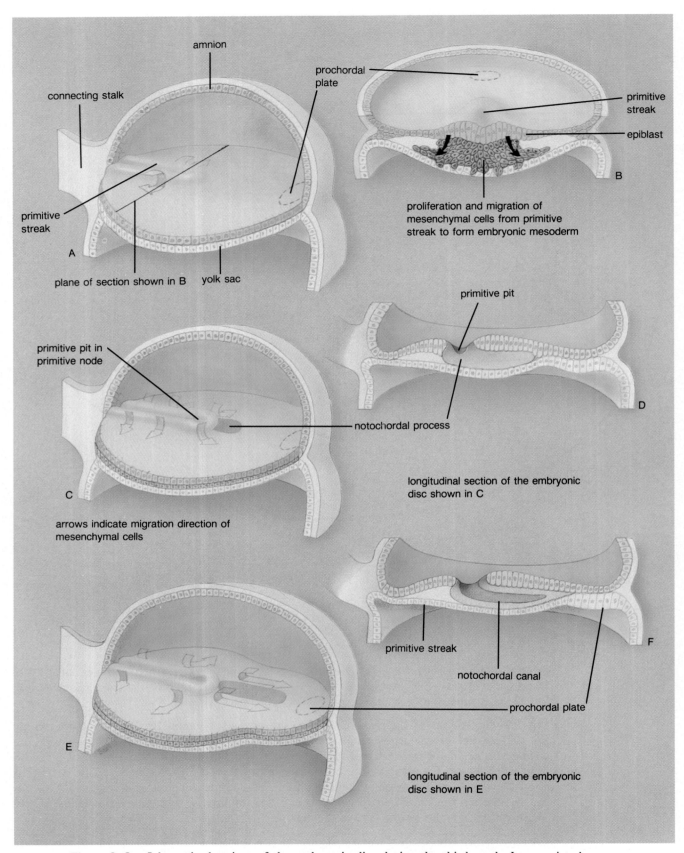

Figure 2-2. Schematic drawings of the embryonic disc during the third week. Its associated membranes (amnion and yolk sac) have been cut away to show the developmental features of the embryonic disc. In *B*, note that mesenchyme (embryonic connective tissue) arises from the primitive streak. The prochordal plate, an organizer of the head region, indicates the future site of the mouth. The notochordal process is soon transformed into the notochord (Fig. 2–3), which forms the axis of the embryo.

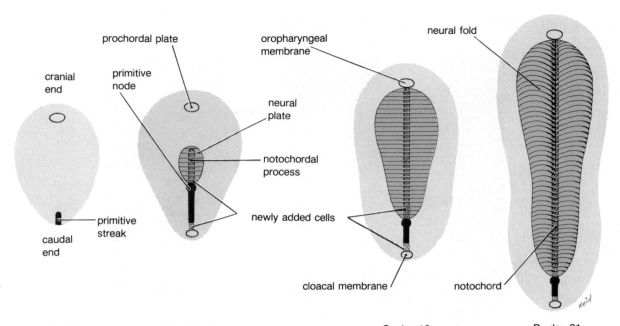

A. day 15   B. day 17   C. day 18   D. day 21

Figure 2–3. Sketches of dorsal views of the embryonic disc (15 to 21 days) showing how it lengthens and changes shape. The neural folds fuse to form the neural tube, the primordium of the central nervous system. The primitive streak lengthens by addition of cells at its caudal end. The primitive streak actively forms mesoderm until the end of the fourth week; thereafter, production of mesoderm slows down. The primitive streak diminishes in relative size and usually becomes an insignificant structure in the sacrococcygeal region of the embryo and normally disappears. (From Moore KL and Persaud TVN: *The Developing Human,* ed 5. Philadelphia, WB Saunders, 1993.)

Figure 2–4. Female infant with a large sacrococcygeal teratoma that developed from remnants of the primitive streak. The tumor, a neoplasm made up of several different types of tissue, was surgically removed. About 75 per cent of infants with these tumors are female; the reason for this preponderance is unknown (Courtesy of Dr. A.E. Chudley, Children's Centre, Winnipeg, Canada).

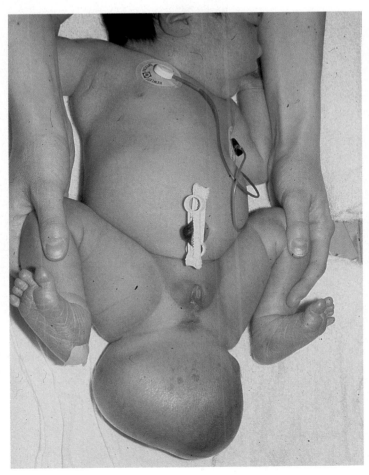

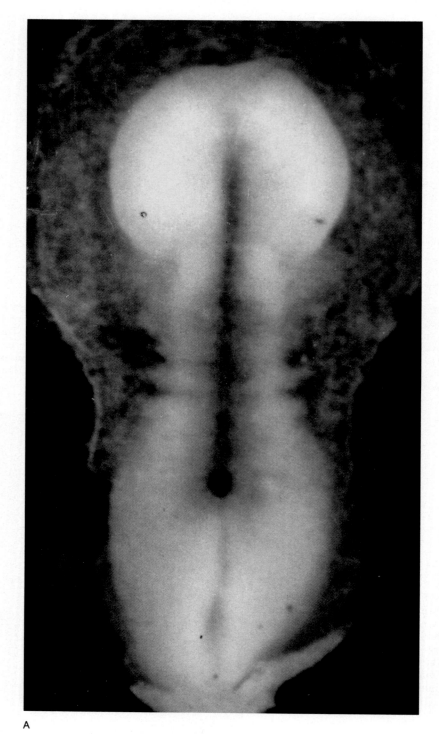

A

Figure 2-5. *A,* Dorsal view of an embryo during the early period of somite formation. Carnegie stage 9, about 19 days. Most of the amnion has been removed to expose the embryo. *B,* Diagram indicating the structures shown in *A.* The mesoderm along the axis of the embryo (paraxial mesoderm) has just begun to divide to produce somites, the primordia of the dermis, subcutaneous tissue, musculature, and cartilage and bones of the axial skeleton.

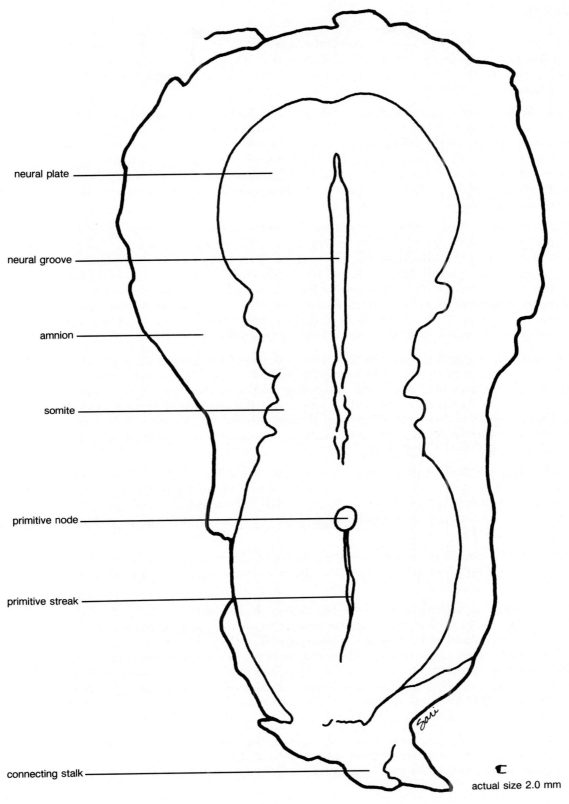

neural plate

neural groove

amnion

somite

primitive node

primitive streak

connecting stalk

actual size 2.0 mm

B

Figure 2–5. *Continued.*

THE FOURTH WEEK

At the beginning of the fourth week, the embryo is almost straight, and the **somites** form conspicuous surface elevations (Figs. 2–6 and 2–7). A significant event occurring during the fourth week is folding of the flat trilaminar embryonic disc into an embryo (Figs. 2–6*F*, 2–8, and 2–9).

Embryonic folding occurs in both the median and horizontal planes and results from the rapid growth of the embryo, particularly the central nervous system (CNS), i.e., the brain and spinal cord. Folding of the embryo produces *head and tail folds* that result in the cranial and caudal regions moving ventrally (Fig. 2–10). Folding of the embryo in the horizontal plane produces right and left *lateral folds.* Each fold moves toward the median plane, rolling the embryonic disc ventrally and forming a roughly cylindrical embryo (Fig. 2–11; see also Fig. 6–2).

Fusion of the neural folds in the fourth week forms the **neural tube** (Figs. 2–6 and 2–7), the primordium of the CNS. The *neural folds* at the cranial end of the embryo thicken to form the primordium of the brain (Figs. 2–6 to 2–8). By the middle of the fourth week, the neural tube is formed opposite the somites, but it is widely open at the rostral and caudal **neuropores** (Figs. 2–6 and 2–8). The rostral (anterior) neuropore normally closes on days 24 to 26 and the caudal (posterior) neuropore closes by 28 days. The embryo is now slightly curved due to the head and tail folds, and the heart produces a large ventral prominence (Figs. 2–9).

As the neural tube separates from the surface ectoderm, the **neural crest** forms (Fig. 2–6*E*). It forms an irregular, flattened cellular mass between the neural tube and the surface ectoderm. *Neural crest cells* migrating from this crest give rise to spinal ganglia (dorsal root ganglia), autonomic ganglia, and the ganglia of certain cranial nerves. These cells also form the sheaths of peripheral nerves, the meninges covering the CNS, and various other structures, such as skeletal and muscular components in the head and neck (see Chapter 7).

Three pairs of *branchial or pharyngeal arches* are visible by 26 days (Figs. 2–10 and 2–11), and the rostral neuropore is closed. Failure of this neuropore to close results in meroanencephaly (anencephaly [see Fig. 13–12]) or meningoencephalocele (see Fig. 13–10). Failure of the caudal neuropore to close results in *spina bifida cystica* (see Fig. 13–15).

The *forebrain* now produces a prominent elevation of the head, and folding of the embryo in the median plane has given the embryo a characteristic C-shaped curvature.

Limb buds appear as swellings on the ventrolateral body walls by the end of the fourth week (Fig. 2–11). The *otic pits,* the primordia of the internal ears, are also clearly visible. Four pairs of **branchial (or pharyngeal) arches** are also visible by the end of the fourth week (Fig. 2–11). They are involved with the formation of the head and neck (see Chapter 7). Ectodermal thickenings called *lens placodes,* indicating the future lenses of the eyes, are visible on the sides of the head. By the end of the fourth week, the *attenuated tail* is a characteristic feature (Figs. 2–11 and 2–12).

Because the CNS, heart, limbs, eyes, and ears are in their critical stages of development during the fourth week, teratogenic agents may cause severe congenital anomalies (e.g., absence of the limbs and congenital cataracts; see Chapter 5).

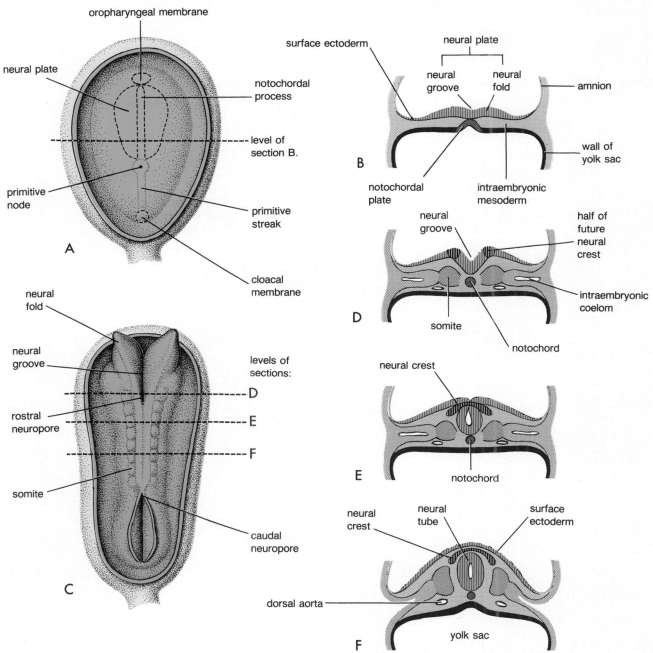

Figure 2-6. Diagrams illustrating folding of the neural plate into the neural tube and formation of the neural crest. *A,* Dorsal view of an embryo of about 18 days, exposed by removing the amnion. *B,* Transverse section of this embryo, showing the neural plate and early development of the neural groove. The developing notochord is also shown. *C,* Dorsal view of an embryo of about 22 days. The neural folds have fused opposite the somites but are widely spread out at both ends of the embryo. The rostral and caudal neuropores are indicated. *D* to *F,* Transverse sections of this embryo at the levels shown in *C,* illustrating formation of the neural tube and its detachment from the surface ectoderm. Note that some neuroectodermal cells are not included in the neural tube but remain between it and the surface ectoderm as the neural crest. Neural crest cells are the major source of connective tissue components, including cartilage, bone, and ligaments of the orofacial region. (From Moore KL and Persaud TVN: *The Developing Human,* ed 5. Philadelphia, WB Saunders, 1993.)

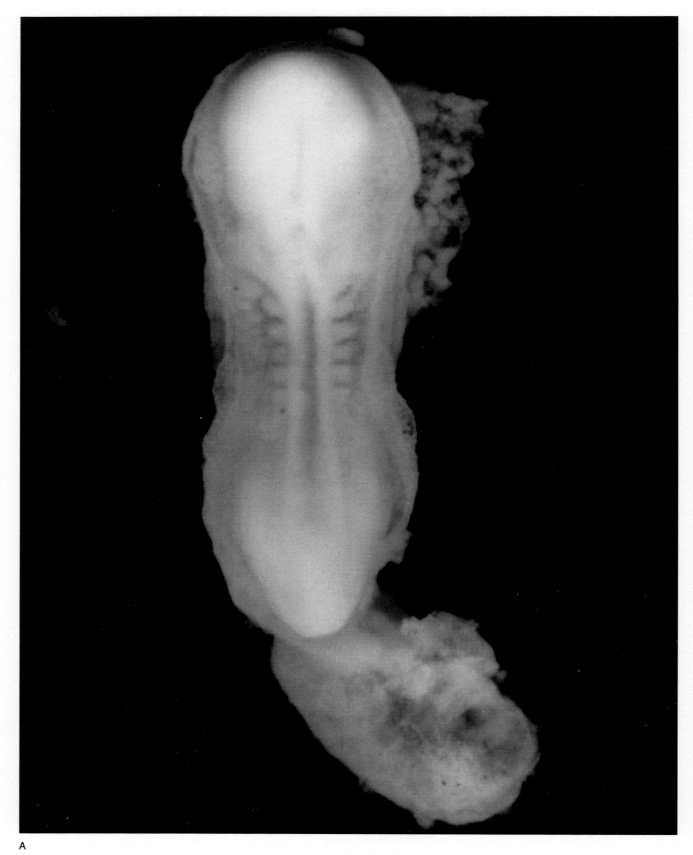

A

Figure 2-7. *A,* Dorsal view of a four-somite embryo at Carnegie stage 10, about 21 days. *B,* Diagram indicating the structures shown in *A.* Most of the amniotic and chorionic sacs have been cut away to expose the embryo. Observe the neural folds and the deep neural groove. The neural folds in the cranial region have thickened to form the primordium of the brain.

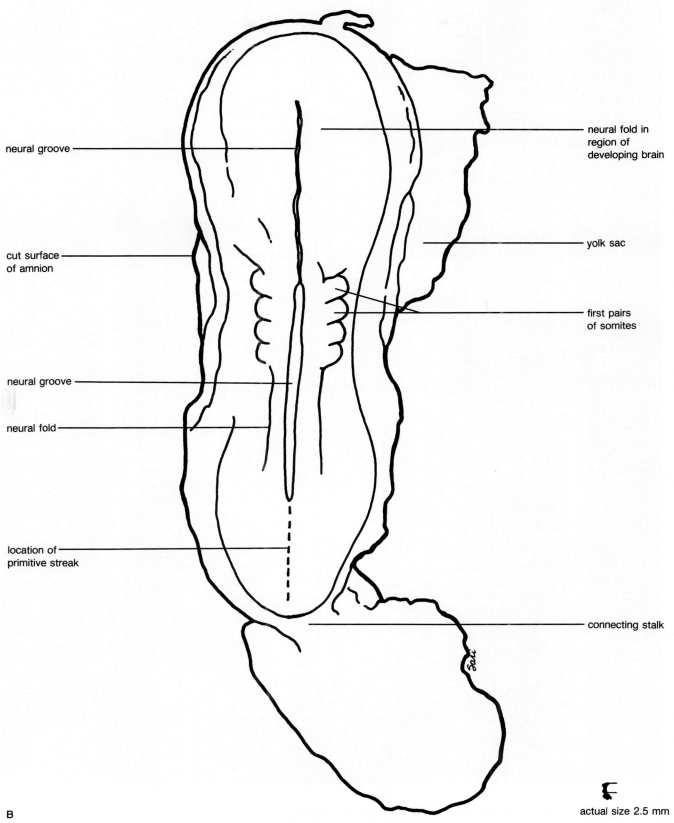

neural groove

cut surface
of amnion

neural groove

neural fold

location of
primitive streak

neural fold in
region of
developing brain

yolk sac

first pairs
of somites

connecting stalk

actual size 2.5 mm

B

Figure 2-7. *Continued.*

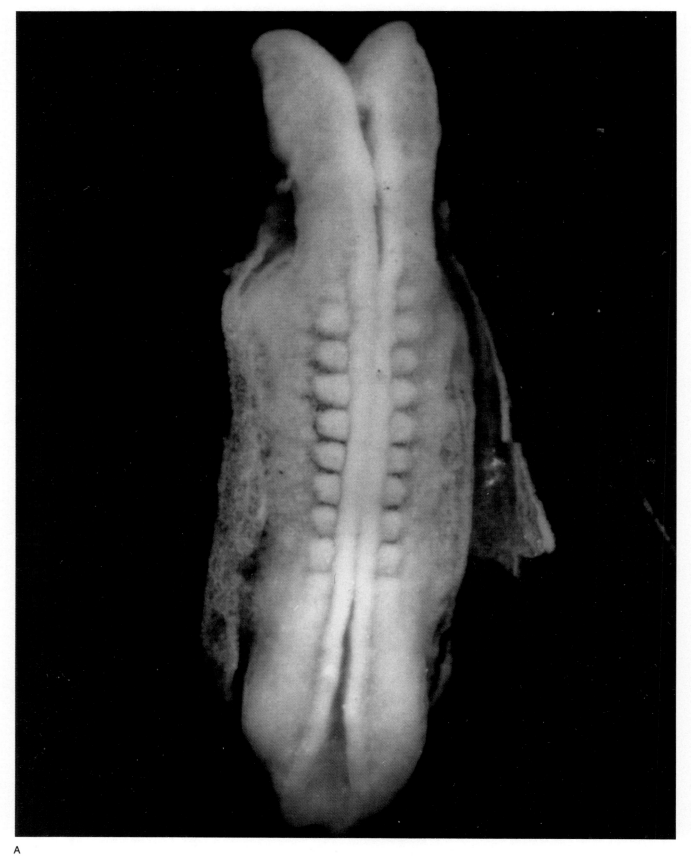

A

Figure 2–8. *A,* Dorsal view of an eight-somite embryo at Carnegie stage 10, about 22 days. *B,* Diagram indicating the structures shown in *A.* The neural folds have fused opposite the somites to form the neural tube (primordium of the spinal cord in this region). The neural tube is in open communication with the amniotic cavity at the cranial and caudal ends by way of the rostral and caudal neuropores, respectively.

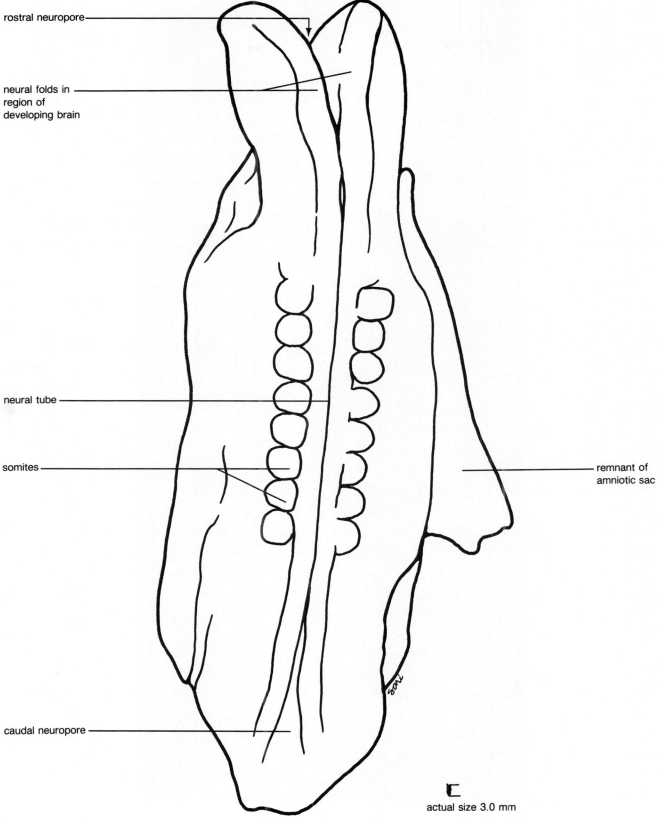

rostral neuropore

neural folds in
region of
developing brain

neural tube

somites

remnant of
amniotic sac

caudal neuropore

actual size 3.0 mm

B

Figure 2–8. *Continued.*

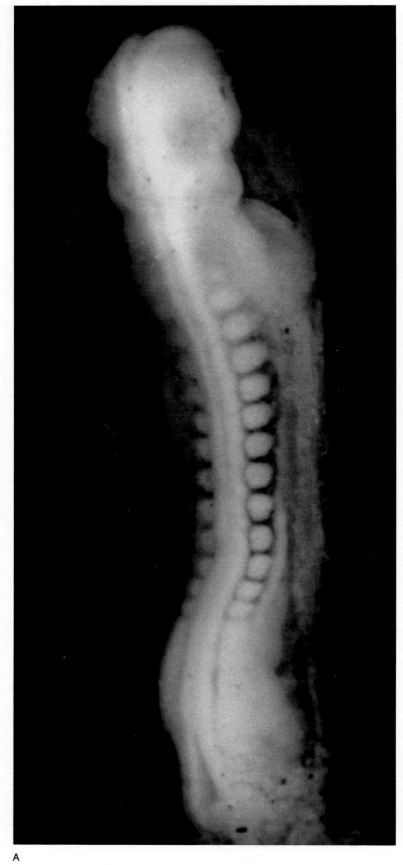

A

Figure 2–9. *A,* Dorsal view of a 13-somite embryo at Carnegie stage 11, about 24 days. *B,* Diagram indicating the structures shown in *A.* The embryo is curved due to folding at the cranial and caudal ends. The rostral neuropore is almost closed, but the caudal neuropore is widely open.

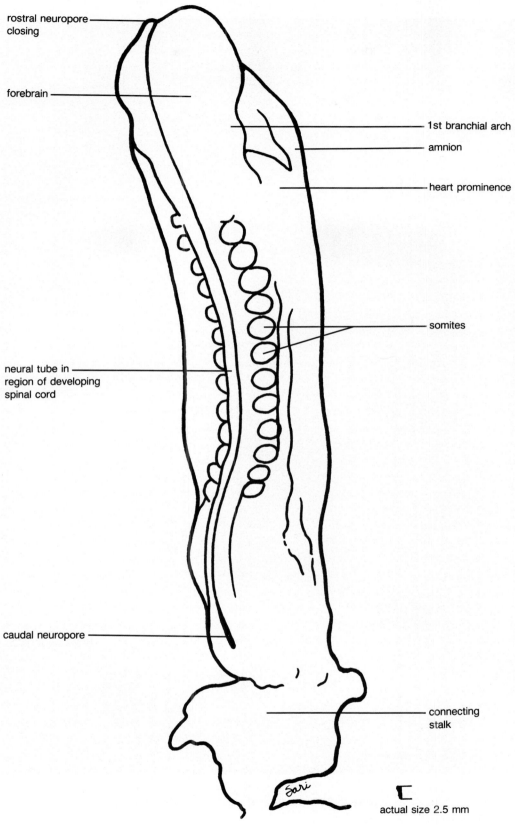

rostral neuropore closing

forebrain

1st branchial arch

amnion

heart prominence

somites

neural tube in region of developing spinal cord

caudal neuropore

connecting stalk

actual size 2.5 mm

B

Figure 2–9. *Continued.*

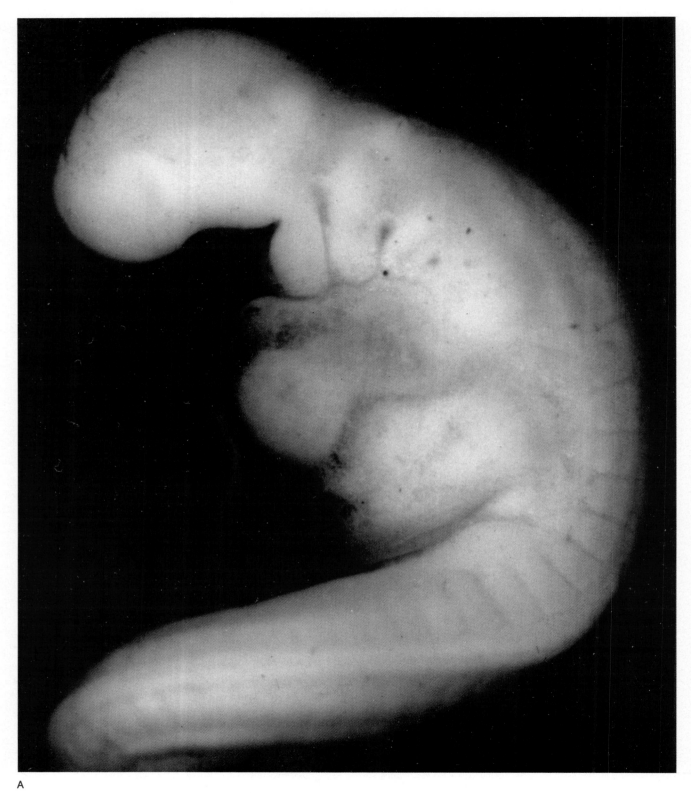

A

Figure 2–10. *See legend on the following page.*

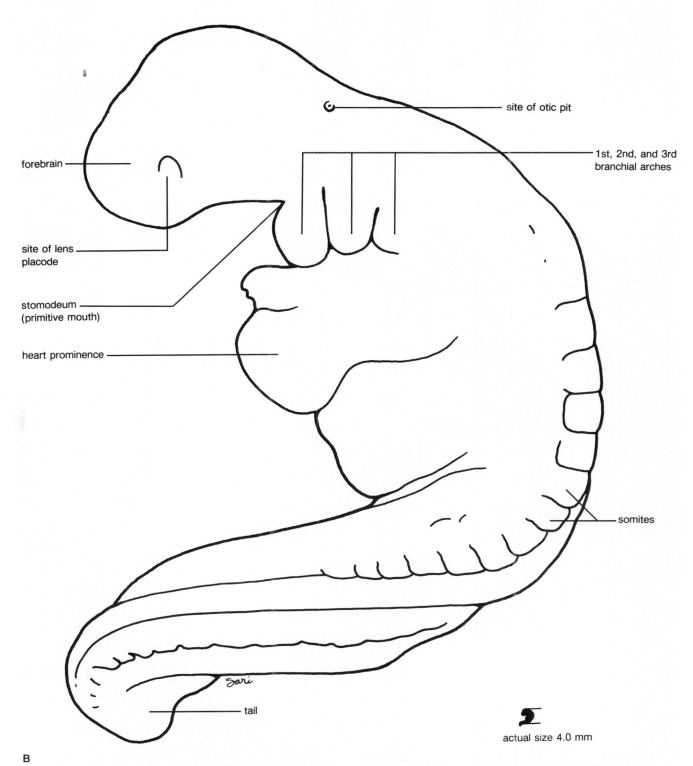

forebrain ———

site of otic pit

1st, 2nd, and 3rd
branchial arches

site of lens
placode

stomodeum
(primitive mouth)

heart prominence ———

somites

tail

actual size 4.0 mm

B

Figure 2–10. *A*, Lateral view of a 27-somite embryo at Carnegie stage 12, about 26 days. *B*, Diagram indicating the structures shown in *A*. Not all the somites are visible in this photograph. The rostral neuropore is closed and three pairs of branchial (pharyngeal) arches are present. The mandibular prominence of the first arch (primordium of the lower jaw) forms the caudal boundary of the stomodeum (primordium of the mouth). The embryo is very curved, especially its long tail. Observe the lens placode (primordium of the lens) and the otic pit indicating early development of the internal ear (see Chapter 14). (From Nishimura, H., et al.: Prenatal Development of the Human with Special Reference to Craniofacial Structures: An Atlas. Washington, DC, National Institutes of Health, 1977.)

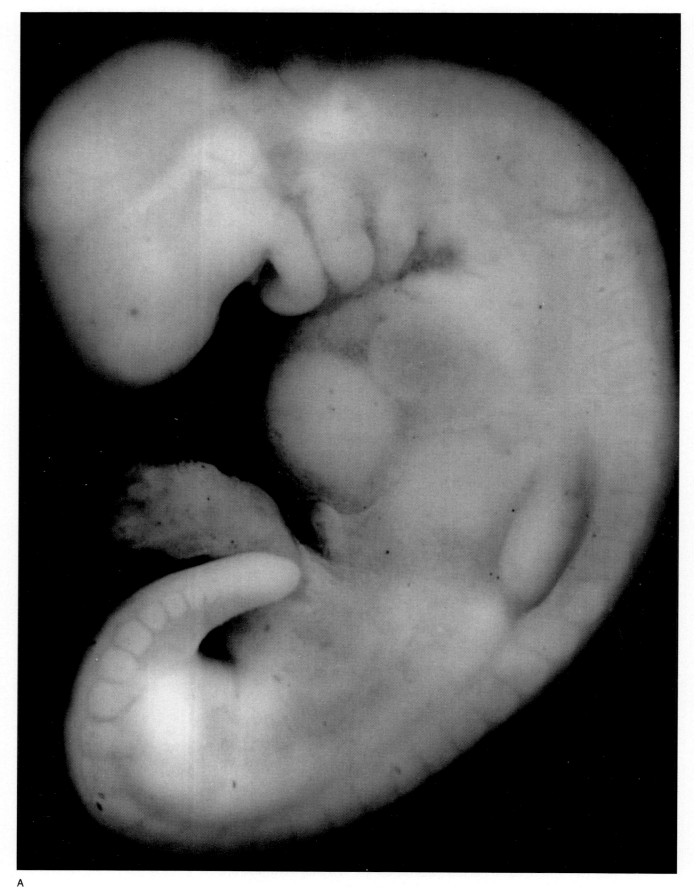

A

Figure 2–11. *See legend on the following page.*

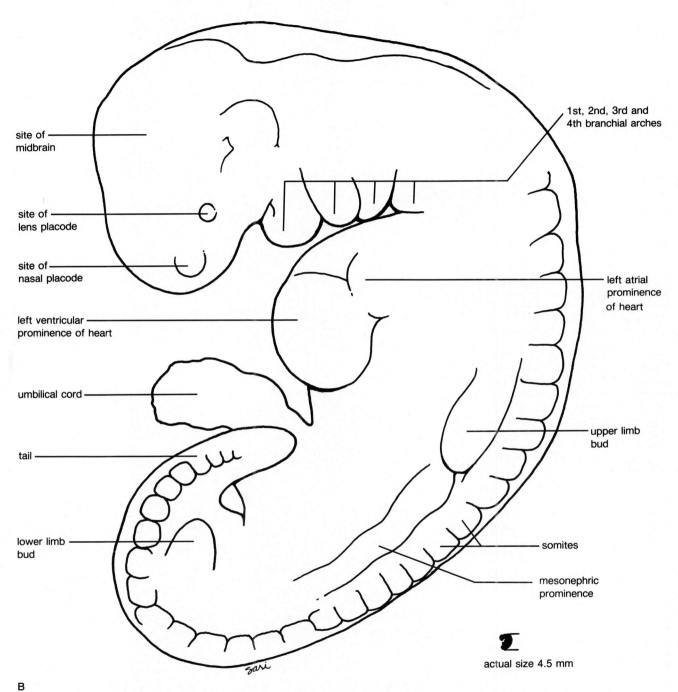

site of
midbrain

1st, 2nd, 3rd and
4th branchial arches

site of
lens placode

site of
nasal placode

left atrial
prominence
of heart

left ventricular
prominence of heart

umbilical cord

tail

upper limb
bud

lower limb
bud

somites

mesonephric
prominence

actual size 4.5 mm

B

Figure 2–11. *A,* Lateral view of an embryo at Carnegie stage 13, about 28 days. *B,* Drawing indicating the structures shown in *A.* The embryo has a characteristic C-shaped curvature, four branchial (pharyngeal) arches, and upper and lower limb buds. The heart is large and its division into a primitive atrium and ventricle is visible. The rostral and caudal neuropores are closed. (From Nishimura, H., et al.: Prenatal Development of the Human with Special Reference to Craniofacial Structures: An Atlas. Washington, DC, National Institutes of Health, 1977.)

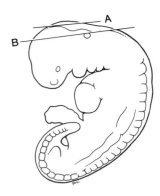

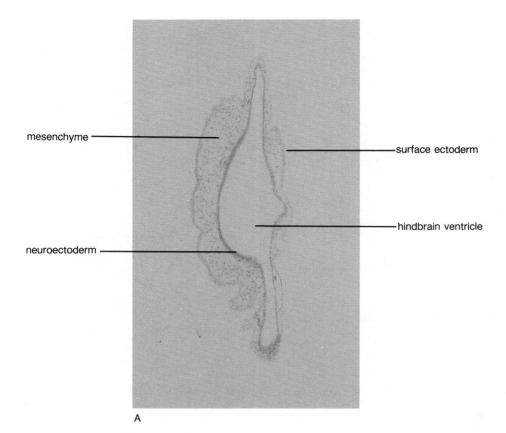

mesenchyme

surface ectoderm

hindbrain ventricle

neuroectoderm

A

Figure 2–12. Selected serial sections of an embryo at Carnegie stage 13, about 28 days. The level of each section is indicated on the small sketch of the embryo. *A,* Section through the thin-walled roof of the hindbrain (rhombencephalon). *B,* Section through the thicker, dorsal part of the hindbrain and the otic vesicles (primordia of the membranous labyrinth of the internal ear).

Legend continues on the following page.

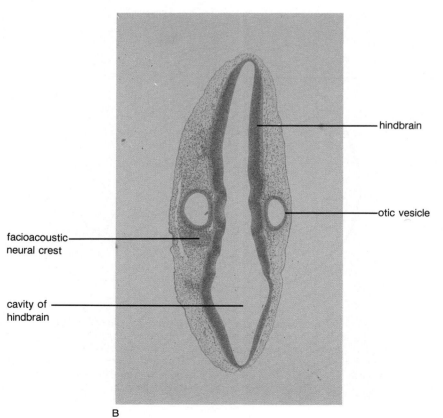

hindbrain

otic vesicle

facioacoustic neural crest

cavity of hindbrain

B

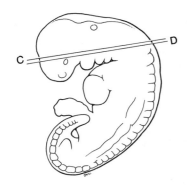

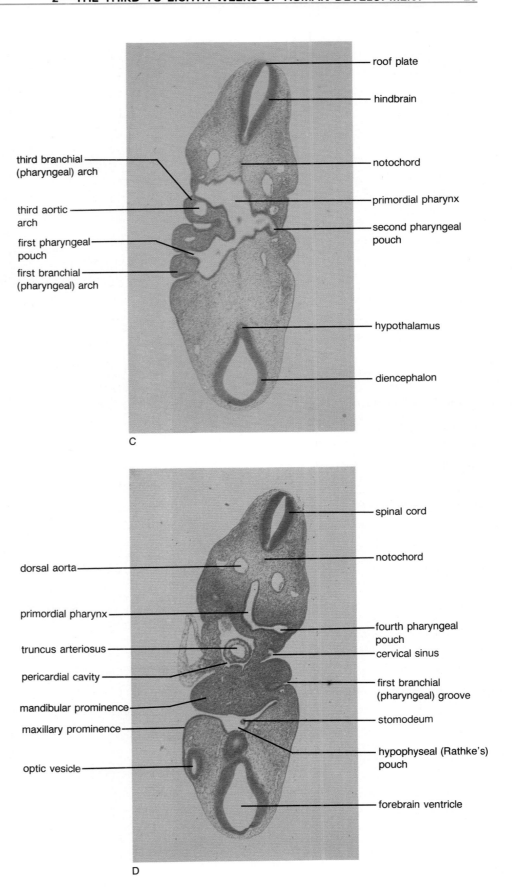

Figure 2-12. *Continued. C,* Section through the diencephalon, hindbrain, and the primordial pharynx. Observe the first three branchial (pharyngeal) arches and the first and second pharyngeal pouches. *D,* Section through the forebrain, spinal cord, primordial pharynx, edge of the optic vesicle, and the truncus arteriosus of the embryonic heart.
Legend continues on the following page.

C labels:
- third branchial (pharyngeal) arch
- third aortic arch
- first pharyngeal pouch
- first branchial (pharyngeal) arch
- roof plate
- hindbrain
- notochord
- primordial pharynx
- second pharyngeal pouch
- hypothalamus
- diencephalon

D labels:
- dorsal aorta
- primordial pharynx
- truncus arteriosus
- pericardial cavity
- mandibular prominence
- maxillary prominence
- optic vesicle
- spinal cord
- notochord
- fourth pharyngeal pouch
- cervical sinus
- first branchial (pharyngeal) groove
- stomodeum
- hypophyseal (Rathke's) pouch
- forebrain ventricle

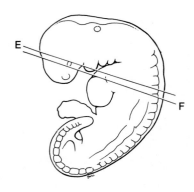

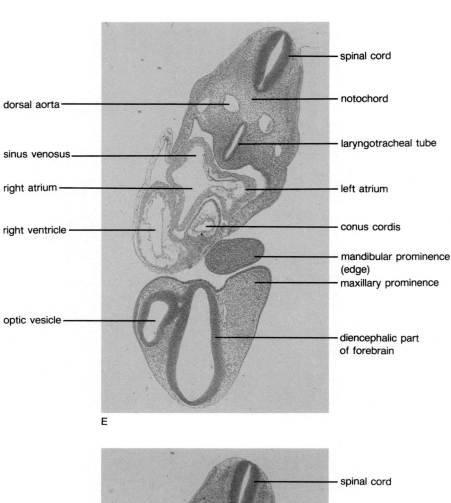

dorsal aorta

sinus venosus

right atrium

right ventricle

optic vesicle

spinal cord

notochord

laryngotracheal tube

left atrium

conus cordis

mandibular prominence (edge)

maxillary prominence

diencephalic part of forebrain

E

Figure 2–12. *Continued. E,* Section through the diencephalon, spinal cord, embryonic heart, and optic vesicle. *F,* Section through the forebrain, spinal cord, heart, esophagus, tracheal bifurcation, and the communication between the forebrain and the optic vesicle. *Legend continues on the following page.*

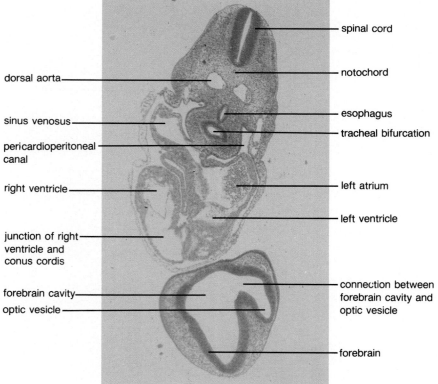

dorsal aorta

sinus venosus

pericardioperitoneal canal

right ventricle

junction of right ventricle and conus cordis

forebrain cavity

optic vesicle

spinal cord

notochord

esophagus

tracheal bifurcation

left atrium

left ventricle

connection between forebrain cavity and optic vesicle

forebrain

F

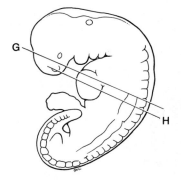

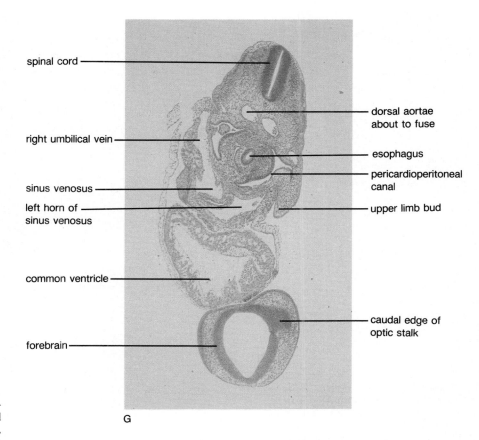

spinal cord

right umbilical vein

sinus venosus

left horn of
sinus venosus

common ventricle

forebrain

dorsal aortae
about to fuse

esophagus

pericardioperitoneal
canal

upper limb bud

caudal edge of
optic stalk

G

Figure 2–12. *Continued. G,* Section through the forebrain, caudal edge of the optic stalk, the heart, and the esophagus. Observe the pericardioperitoneal canal that connects the pericardial and peritoneal cavities (see Chapter 6). *H,* Section through the common ventricle, sinus venosus, upper limb bud, primitive stomach, and spinal cord.

Legend continues on the following page.

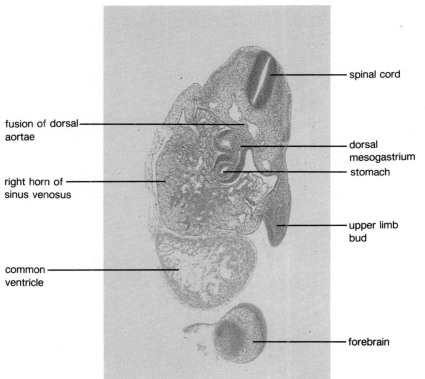

fusion of dorsal
aortae

right horn of
sinus venosus

common
ventricle

spinal cord

dorsal
mesogastrium

stomach

upper limb
bud

forebrain

H

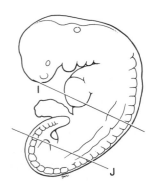

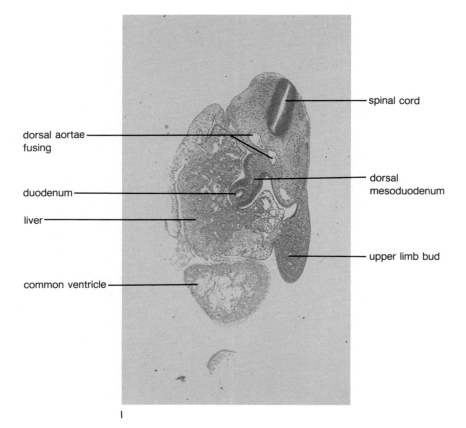

dorsal aortae
fusing

duodenum

liver

common ventricle

spinal cord

dorsal
mesoduodenum

upper limb bud

I

Figure 2–12. *Continued. I,* Section through the common ventricle of the heart, upper limb bud, duodenum, liver, and spinal cord. *J,* Section through the caudal end of the embryo showing the lower limb bud, hindgut, urogenital sinus, and umbilical arteries.

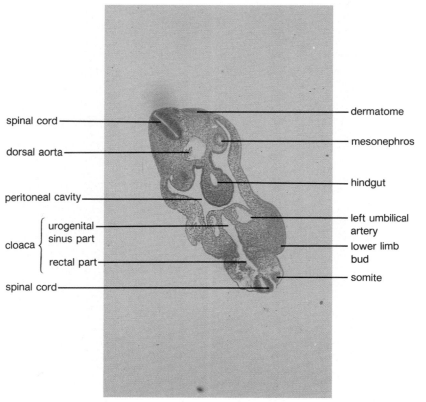

spinal cord

dorsal aorta

peritoneal cavity

cloaca {
  urogenital
  sinus part

  rectal part
}

spinal cord

dermatome

mesonephros

hindgut

left umbilical
artery

lower limb
bud

somite

J

THE FIFTH TO EIGHTH WEEKS

The Fifth Week

Changes in body form are minor during this week compared with those that occurred during the fourth week, but growth of the head exceeds that of other regions due to rapid development of the brain (Figs. 2–13, 2–14A, and 2–15). The face soon contacts the heart prominence. The second branchial (pharyngeal) arch has overgrown the third and fourth arches, forming an ectodermal depression known as the **cervical sinus** (Fig. 2–15). The distal ends of the upper limbs become paddle-shaped. It has been reported that embryos show spontaneous movements in the fifth week, such as twitching of the trunk and limbs.

The Sixth Week

The upper limbs show rapid regional differentiation during the sixth week (Figs. 2–16 to 2–19). The elbow and wrist regions are clearly identifiable and **digital rays,** indicating the future digits, are clearly visible by the end of the sixth week (Fig. 2–19). Development of the lower limbs occurs about two days later than that of the upper limbs (Fig. 2–13). Six small swellings develop around the branchial (pharyngeal) groove between the first two branchial arches (Figs. 2–17 and 2–19). This groove becomes the *external acoustic meatus* and the swellings around it fuse to form the auricle (pinna) of the external ear. Largely because *retinal pigment* has formed, the eye is now obvious (Figs. 2–14B, 2–17, and 2–19). The head is now much larger relative to the trunk and is more bent over the **heart prominence.** This head position results from bending of the brain in the cervical region.

The Seventh and Eighth Weeks

The limbs undergo considerable change during the seventh week (Figs. 2–20 and 2–21). Notches appear between the digital rays in the hand plates, clearly indicating the future digits. At the beginning of the eighth week, the digits of the hand are short and noticeably webbed (Fig. 2–22). Notches are now clearly visible between the digital rays of the feet; and the tail is still present but stubby (Fig. 2–22). The **scalp vascular plexus** soon appears and forms a characteristic band around the head (Figs. 2–22 to 2–24). By the end of the eighth week, all regions of the limbs are apparent, and the digits have lengthened and are separated (Figs. 2–13, 2–14C, and 2–25). *Purposeful limb movements* first occur during the eighth week. All evidence of the tail disappears by the end of the eighth week. The scalp vascular plexus is now located near the vertex of the head (Fig. 2–25).

By the end of the eighth week, the embryo has distinct human characteristics; however, the head is still disproportionately large, constituting almost half of the embryo. The neck region is established and the eyelids are more obvious. Early in the eighth week the eyes are open but, toward the end of the week, the eyelids move toward each other. The auricles of the external ears begin to assume their final shape but are still low-set on the head. Although sex differences exist in the appearance of the external genitalia (Fig. 2–26), they are not distinct enough to permit accurate sexual identification by laypeople.

METHODS OF MEASURING EMBRYOS

Because embryos early in the fourth week are straight, measurements of them indicate the greatest length (GL). The sitting height, or *crown-rump length* (CRL), is most frequently used for older embryos. Standing height, or crown-heel length (CHL), is sometimes measured for 8-week-old embryos (Table 2–1). To estimate the age of aborted embryos, the *Carnegie Staging System* is used. It is based on morphologic developmental landmarks of the embryo (O'Rahilly and Müller, 1987, 1992). The size of an embryo in a pregnant woman can be estimated using ultrasound measurements (see Chapter 4). *Transvaginal sonographs* permit an earlier and more accurate measurement of CRL in early pregnancy.

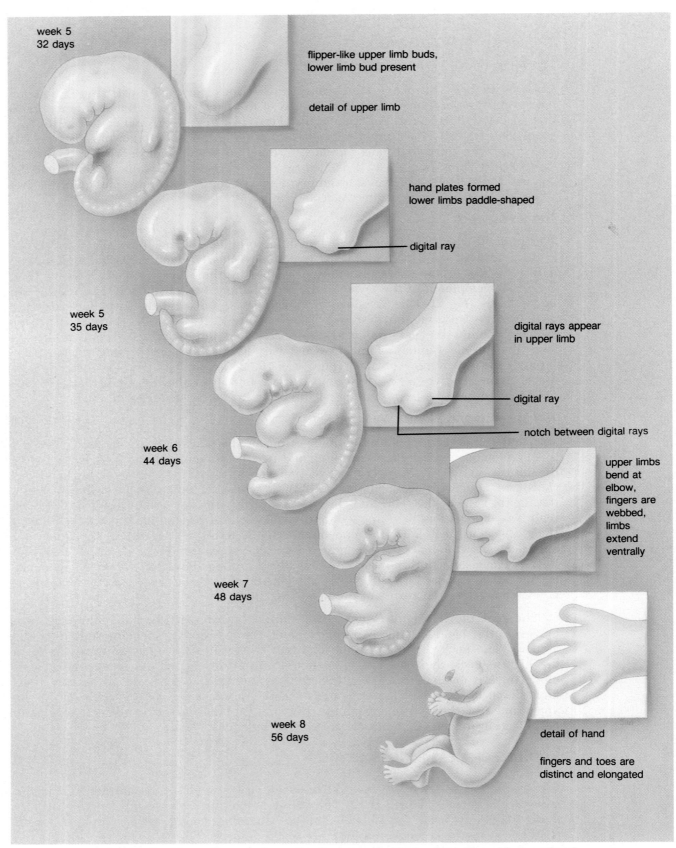

week 5
32 days

flipper-like upper limb buds,
lower limb bud present

detail of upper limb

hand plates formed
lower limbs paddle-shaped

digital ray

week 5
35 days

digital rays appear
in upper limb

digital ray

notch between digital rays

week 6
44 days

upper limbs
bend at
elbow,
fingers are
webbed,
limbs
extend
ventrally

week 7
48 days

week 8
56 days

detail of hand

fingers and toes are
distinct and elongated

Figure 2-13. Drawings of lateral views of embryos ranging in age from 32 to 56 days. Development of the upper limbs is highlighted because their appearance is a reliable guide to stages 13 to 23 of development (see Table 2-1 on page 61).

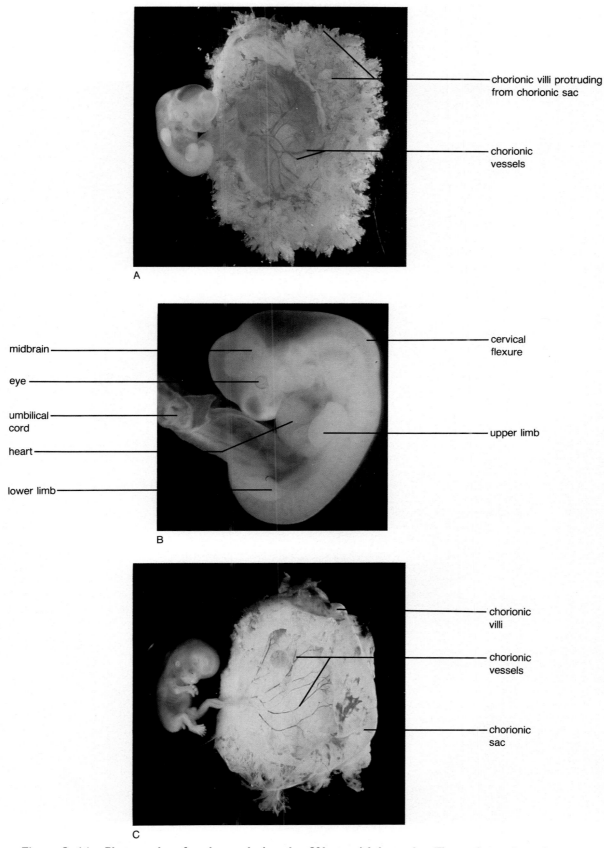

A

chorionic villi protruding
from chorionic sac

chorionic
vessels

midbrain

eye

umbilical
cord

heart

lower limb

B

cervical
flexure

upper limb

C

chorionic
villi

chorionic
vessels

chorionic
sac

Figure 2–14. Photographs of embryos during the fifth to eighth weeks. The embryos have been removed from their amniotic and chorionic sacs. *A,* Lateral view of an embryo at Carnegie stage 14, about 32 days (see also Fig. 2–15). Observe that the chorionic sac is completely covered by chorionic villi. *B,* Lateral view of an embryo at Carnegie stage 15, about 36 days (see also Fig. 2–16). Pigment in the retina makes the eye clearly visible. *C,* Lateral view of an embryo at Carnegie stage 23, about 56 days (see also Figs. 2–25 and 2–26). Observe its human appearance. (From Nishimura, H., et al.: Prenatal Development of the Human with Special Reference to Craniofacial Structures: An Atlas. Washington, DC, National Institutes of Health, 1977.)

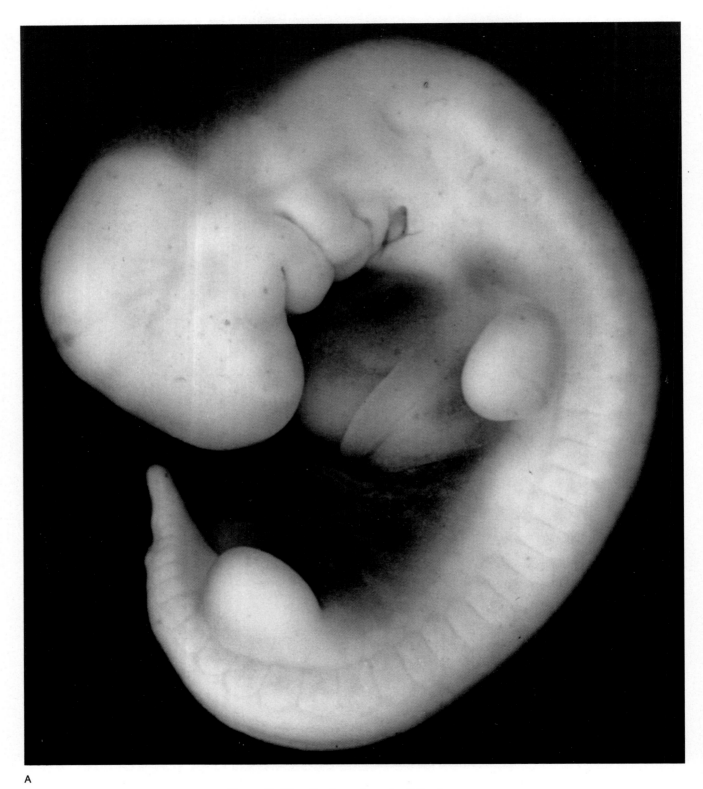

A

Figure 2–15.   *See legend on the following page.*

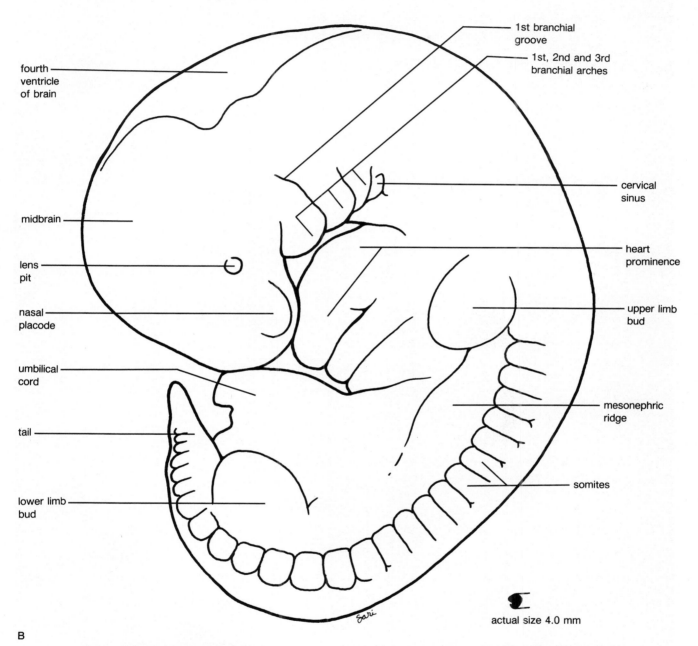

Figure 2–15. *A,* Lateral view of an embryo at Carnegie stage 14, about 32 days. *B,* Drawings indicating the structures shown in *A.* The upper limb buds are paddle-shaped and the lower limb buds are flipperlike. The second branchial (pharyngeal) arch has overgrown the third arch forming an ectoderm depression known as the cervical sinus. The mesonephric ridge indicates the site of the mesonephric kidney, and interim kidney (see Chapter 10). (From Nishimura, H., et al.: Prenatal Development of the Human with Special Reference to Craniofacial Structures: An Atlas. Washington, DC, National Institutes of Health, 1977.)

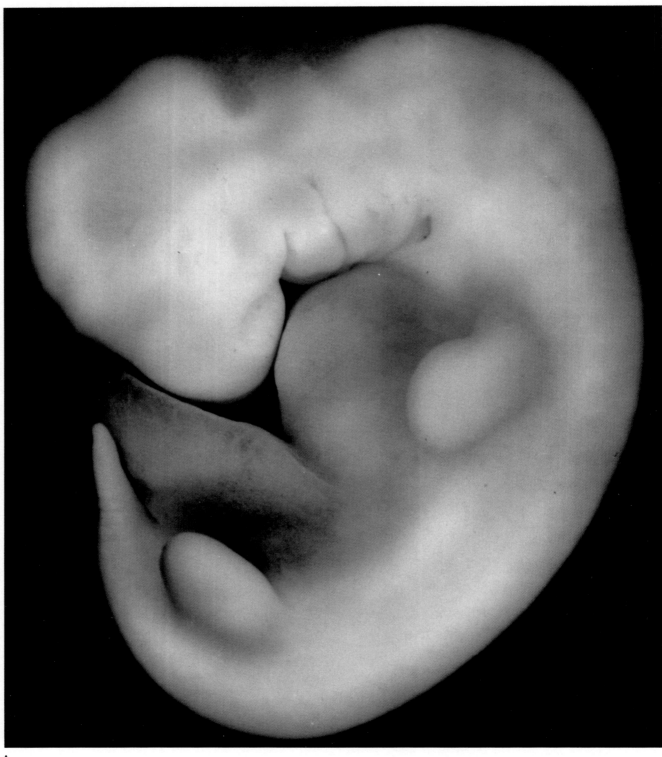

A

Figure 2–16.   *See legend on the following page.*

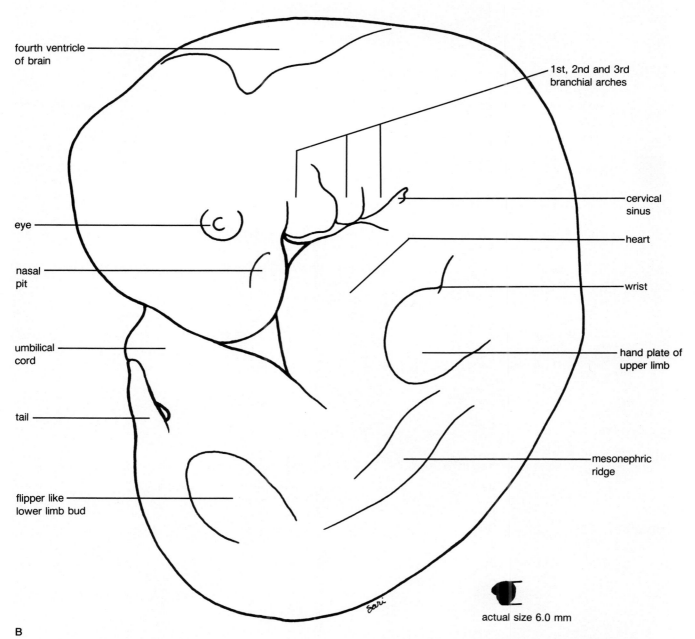

fourth ventricle
of brain

1st, 2nd and 3rd
branchial arches

eye

cervical
sinus

heart

nasal
pit

wrist

umbilical
cord

hand plate of
upper limb

tail

mesonephric
ridge

flipper like
lower limb bud

actual size 6.0 mm

B

Figure 2–16. *A,* Lateral view of an embryo at Carnegie stage 15, about 36 days. *B,* Drawings indicating the structures shown in *A.* The nasal pit (primordium of the nasal aperture and cavity) is now visible, as is the wrist region. The third and fourth branchial (pharyngeal) arches are indistinct due to overgrowth of them by the second arch. The fourth arch is in the cervical sinus. (From Nishimura, H., et al.: Prenatal Development of the Human with Special Reference to Craniofacial Structures: An Atlas. Washington, DC, National Institutes of Health, 1977.)

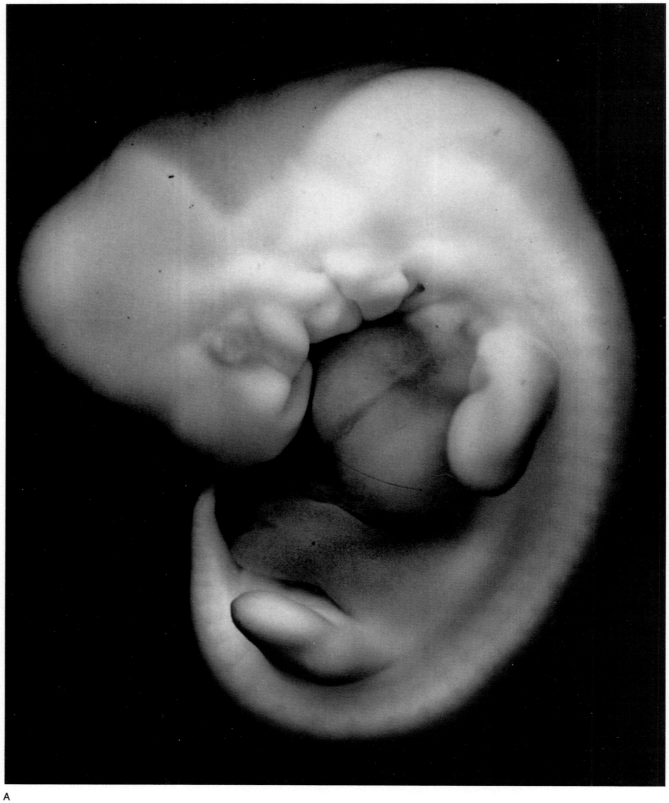

A

Figure 2–17. *See legend on the following page.*

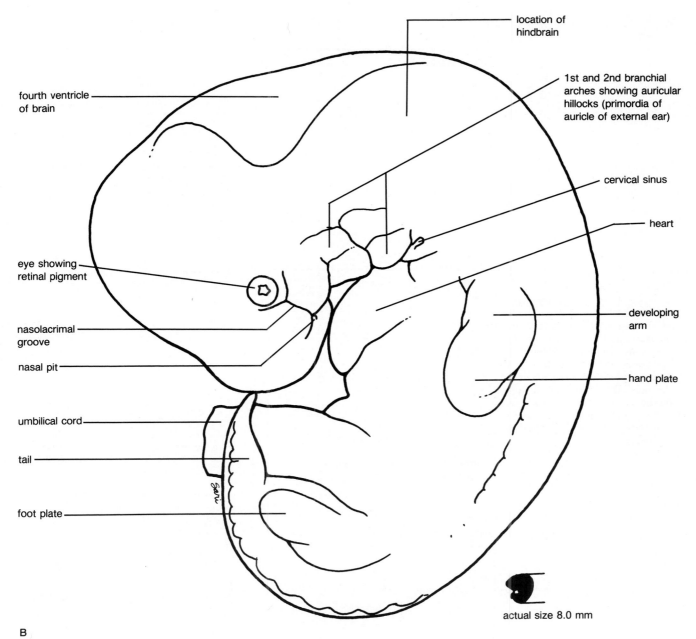

B

Figure 2–17. *A,* Lateral view of an embryo at Carnegie stage 16, about 40 days. *B,* Drawing indicating the structures shown in *A.* The eye is distinct, as are the nasal pit and nasolacrimal groove (primordium of the nasolacrimal duct). The hand plate is more distinct and the foot plate has formed. Small swellings, called auricular hillocks, have developed around the first branchial groove (primordium of the external acoustic meatus). The auricular hillocks will fuse to form the auricle of the external ear (see Chapter 14).

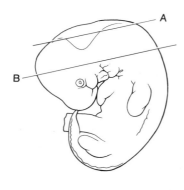

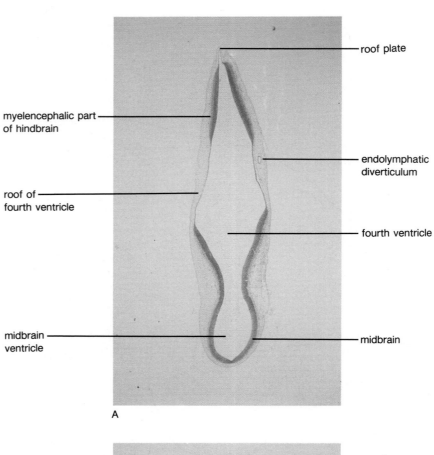

roof plate

myelencephalic part of hindbrain

endolymphatic diverticulum

roof of fourth ventricle

fourth ventricle

midbrain ventricle

midbrain

A

Figure 2–18. Selected serial sections of an embryo at Carnegie stage 16, about 40 days. The level of each section is indicated on the small sketch of the embryo. *A,* Section through the midbrain and the roof of the fourth ventricle. *B,* Section through the cephalic flexure, midbrain, fourth ventricle, otic vesicle, and trigeminal ganglion. *Legend continues on the following page.*

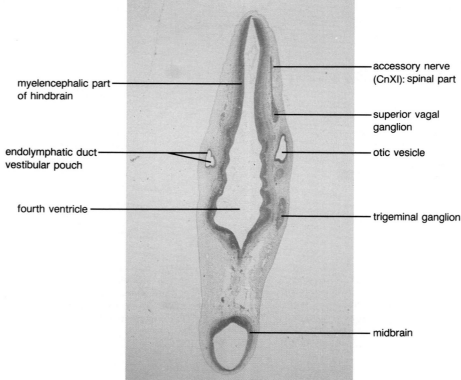

myelencephalic part of hindbrain

accessory nerve (CnXI): spinal part

superior vagal ganglion

endolymphatic duct vestibular pouch

otic vesicle

fourth ventricle

trigeminal ganglion

midbrain

B

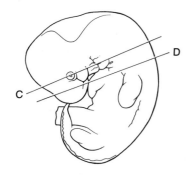

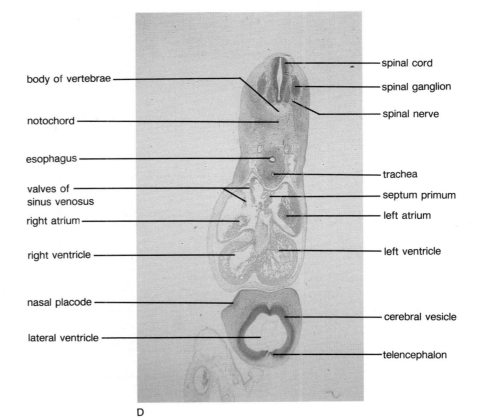

neural canal

sclerotome

notochord

primordial pharynx

hypobranchial eminence

second pharyngeal pouch

first pharyngeal pouch

optic stalk

optic cup

spinal cord

myotome

ventral primary ramus

inferior ganglion of vagus nerve (CnX)

second branchial (pharyngeal) arch

first branchial (pharyngeal) arch

stomodeum (primordial mouth)

lens vesicle

third ventricle

C

Figure 2–18. *Continued. C,* Section through the third ventricle, spinal cord, primordial pharynx, stomodeum (primordial mouth), developing tongue, optic cup, and lens vesicle. Observe the first and second branchial (pharyngeal) arches. *D,* Section through the cerebral vesicle, lateral ventricle, ventricles of the heart, esophagus, and trachea.
Legend continues on the following page.

body of vertebrae

notochord

esophagus

valves of sinus venosus

right atrium

right ventricle

nasal placode

lateral ventricle

spinal cord

spinal ganglion

spinal nerve

trachea

septum primum

left atrium

left ventricle

cerebral vesicle

telencephalon

D

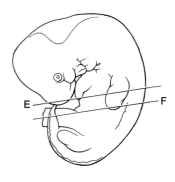

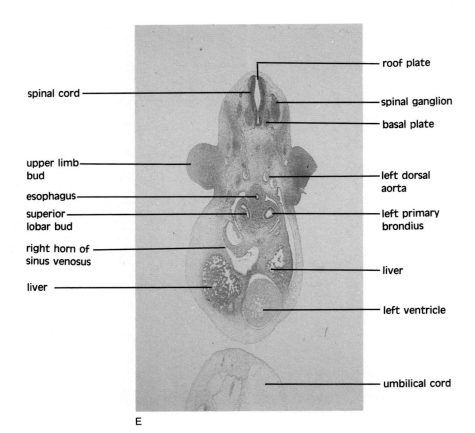

spinal cord — — roof plate

— spinal ganglion

— basal plate

upper limb bud —

— left dorsal aorta

esophagus —

superior lobar bud —

— left primary brondius

right horn of sinus venosus —

— liver

liver —

— left ventricle

— umbilical cord

E

Figure 2–18. *Continued. E,* Section through the liver, left primary bronchus, heart, esophagus, and upper limb bud. *F,* Section through the tail of the embryo, umbilical cord, liver, stomach, mesonephros, upper limb, and spinal cord. *Legend continues on the following page.*

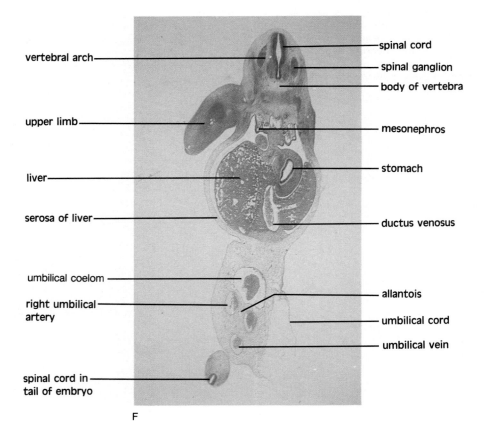

vertebral arch —

— spinal cord

— spinal ganglion

— body of vertebra

upper limb —

— mesonephros

liver —

— stomach

serosa of liver —

— ductus venosus

umbilical coelom —

— allantois

right umbilical artery —

— umbilical cord

— umbilical vein

spinal cord in tail of embryo —

F

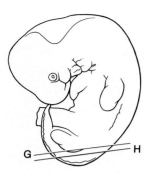

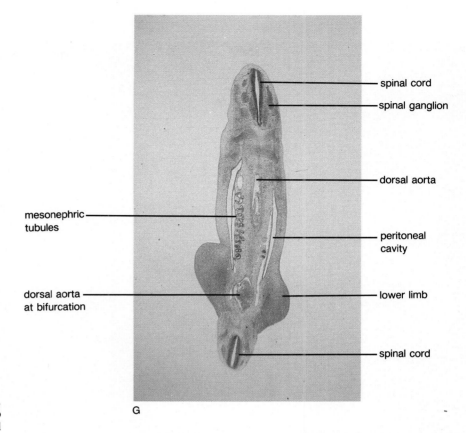

mesonephric tubules

spinal cord

spinal ganglion

dorsal aorta

peritoneal cavity

dorsal aorta at bifurcation

lower limb

spinal cord

G

Figure 2–18. *Continued. G,* Section through the lower limb buds, mesonephros, and spinal cord. *H,* Section through the caudal end of the embryo.

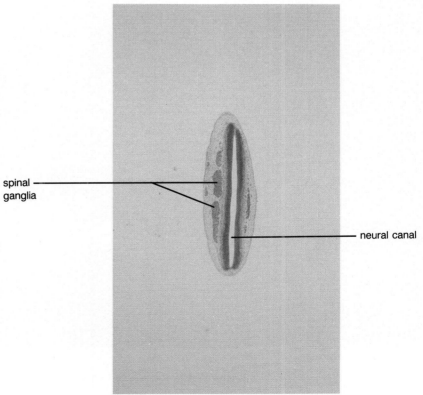

spinal ganglia

neural canal

H

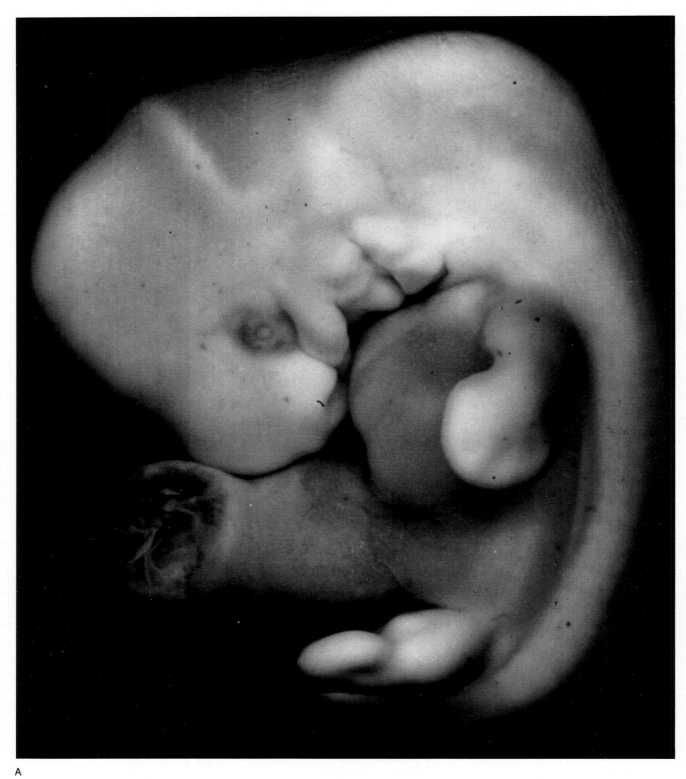

A

Figure 2-19. *See legend on the following page.*

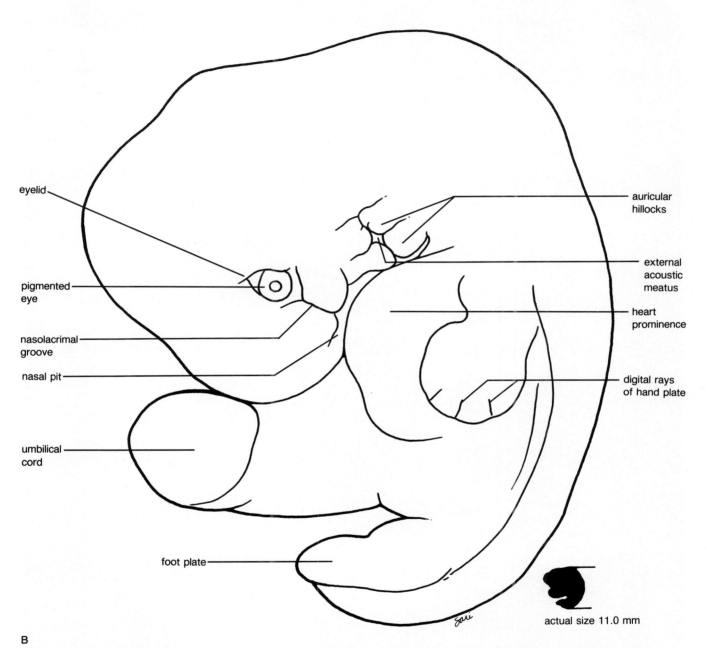

eyelid

pigmented
eye

nasolacrimal
groove

nasal pit

umbilical
cord

foot plate

auricular
hillocks

external
acoustic
meatus

heart
prominence

digital rays
of hand plate

actual size 11.0 mm

B

Figure 2–19. *A,* Lateral view of an embryo at Carnegie stage 17, about 42 days. *B,* Drawing indicating the structures shown in *A.* The eye, auricular hillocks (primordia of external ear), and external acoustic meatus (auditory canal) are now more obvious. Digital rays in the large hand plate, indicating the future site of the digits, are now clearly visible.

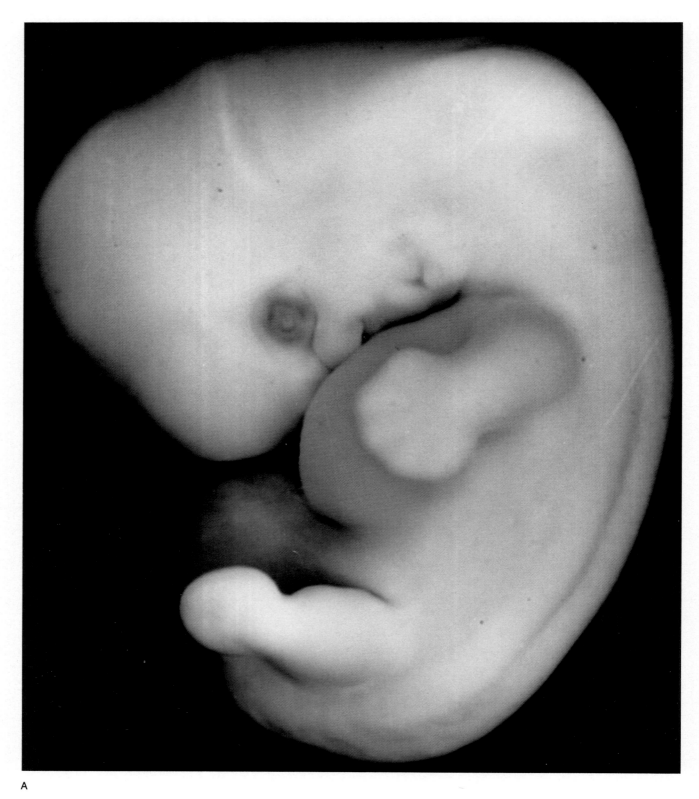

A

Figure 2–20.   *See legend on the following page.*

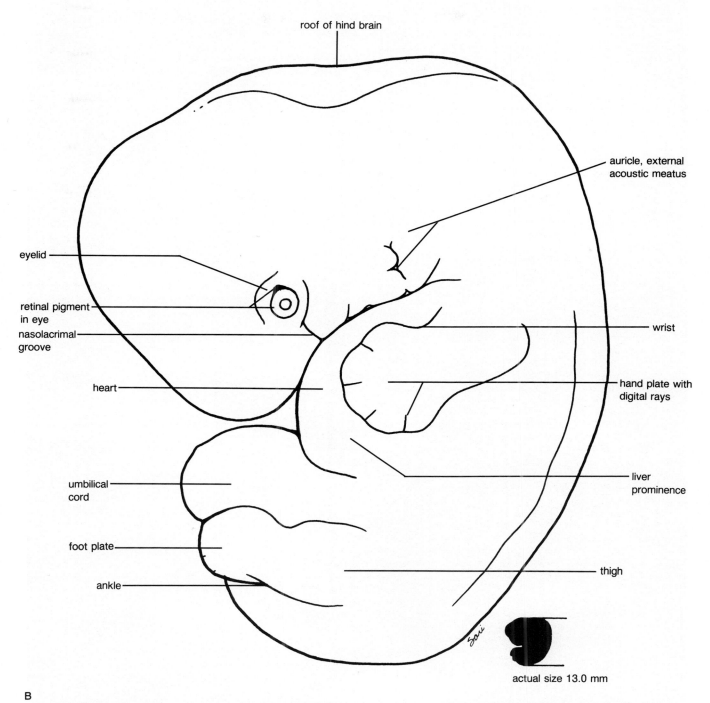

roof of hind brain

auricle, external
acoustic meatus

eyelid

retinal pigment
in eye

nasolacrimal
groove

heart

wrist

hand plate with
digital rays

umbilical
cord

liver
prominence

foot plate

ankle

thigh

actual size 13.0 mm

B

Figure 2-20. *A*, Lateral view of an embryo at Carnegie stage 18, about 44 days. *B*, Drawing indicating the structures shown in *A*. The eye is prominent due to the presence of retinal pigment. The hand plate is very large and the digital rays are distinctive. The foot plate is well formed and the ankle region is visible. The auricle of the external ear is now distinguishable. The branchial (pharyngeal) arches are no longer distinct and the cervical sinus (visible in Fig. 2-15) has disappeared. (From Nishimura, H., et al.: Prenatal Development of the Human with Special Reference to Craniofacial Structures: An Atlas. Washington, DC, National Institutes of Health, 1977.)

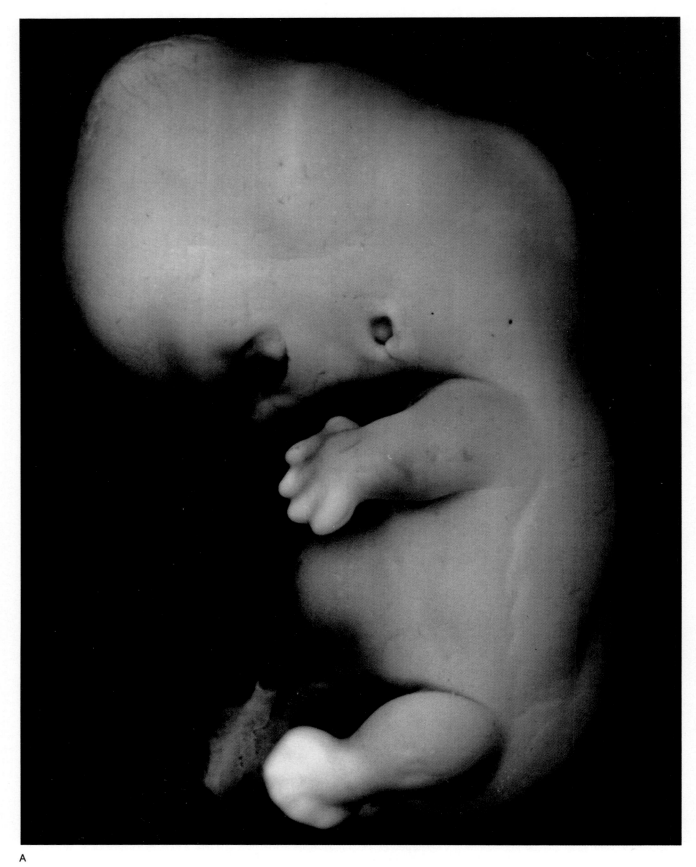

A

Figure 2–21. *See legend on the following page.*

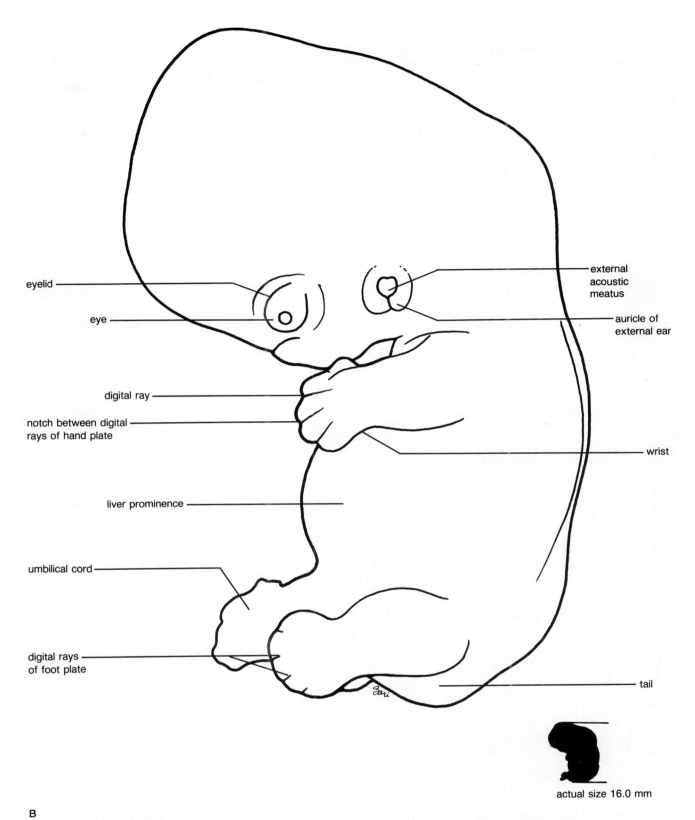

eyelid

eye

digital ray

notch between digital
rays of hand plate

liver prominence

umbilical cord

digital rays
of foot plate

external
acoustic
meatus

auricle of
external ear

wrist

tail

actual size 16.0 mm

B

Figure 2–21. *A,* Lateral view of an embryo at Carnegie stage 19, about 48 days. *B,* Drawing indicating the structures shown in *A.* The notches between the digital rays in the hand clearly indicate the developing digits. The auricle and external acoustic meatus are now clearly visible. Note the low position of the ear at this stage. Digital rays are now visible in the foot plate. The prominence of the abdomen is caused mainly by the large size of the liver.

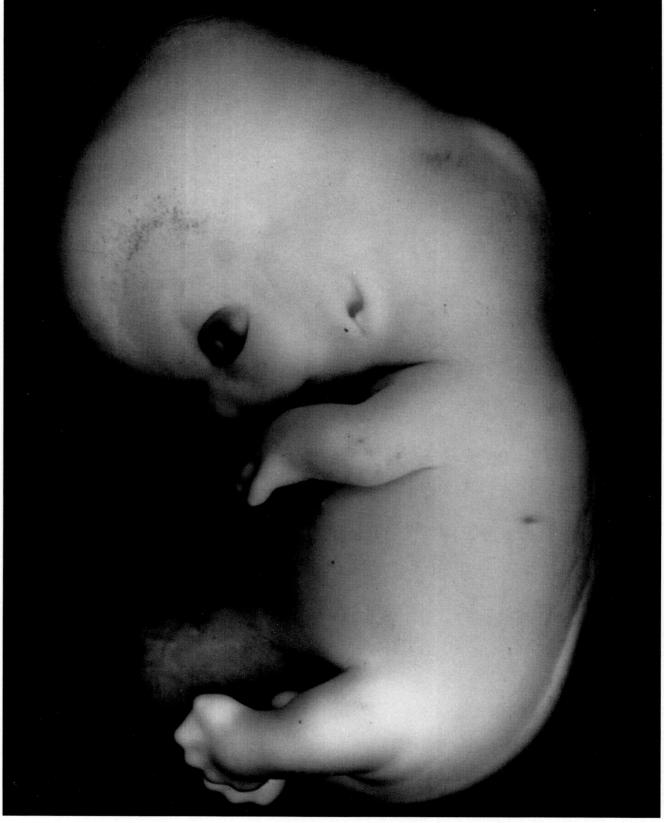

A

Figure 2–22. *See legend on the following page.*

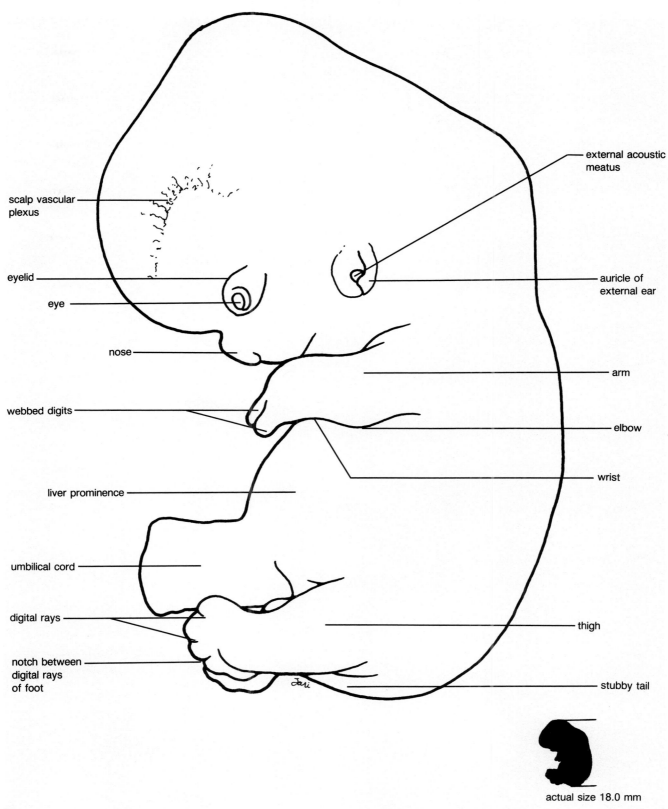

B

Figure 2–22. *A,* Lateral view of an embryo at Carnegie stage 20, about 51 days. *B,* Drawing indicating the structures shown in *A.* The limbs now extend ventrally. The fingers are well formed but are short and webbed. The upper limb is bent at the elbow. Notches have now appeared between the digital rays of the foot. The scalp vascular plexus is now visible. A stubby tail is still present. (From Nishimura, H., et al.: Prenatal Development of the Human with Special Reference to Craniofacial Structures: An Atlas. Washington, DC, National Institutes of Health, 1977.)

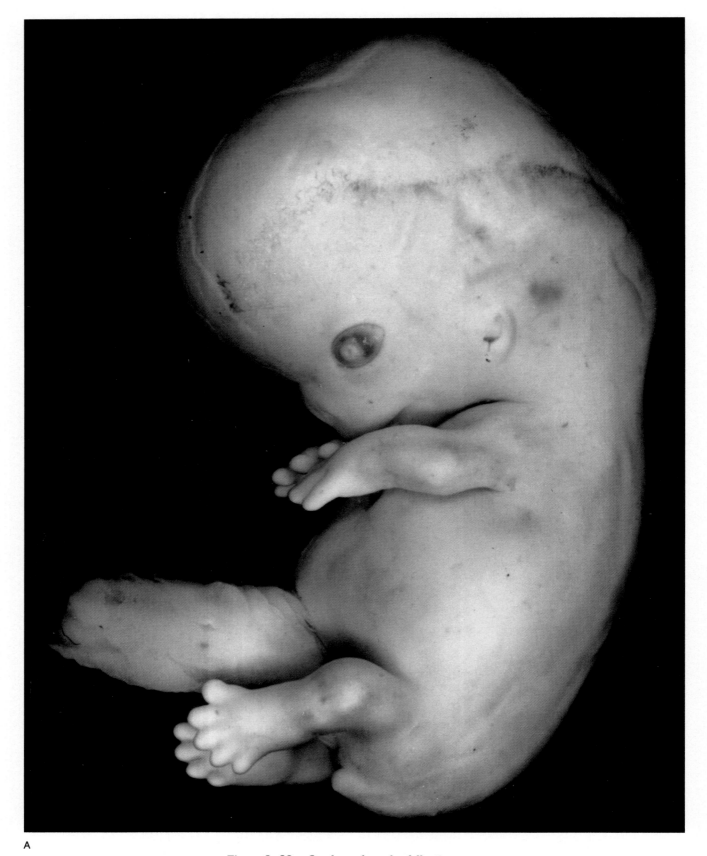

A

Figure 2–23.   *See legend on the following page.*

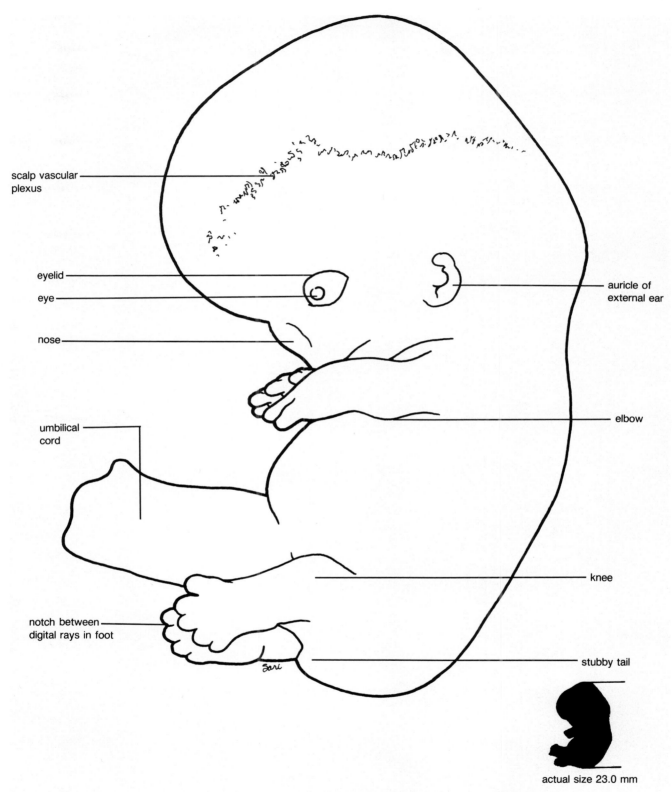

scalp vascular plexus

eyelid

eye

nose

umbilical cord

notch between digital rays in foot

auricle of external ear

elbow

knee

stubby tail

actual size 23.0 mm

B

Figure 2–23. *A,* Lateral view of an embryo at Carnegie stage 21, about 52 days. *B,* Drawing indicating the structures shown in *A.* The fingers are separated and the toes are beginning to separate. Note that the feet are fan-shaped and that the tail is very short. The scalp vascular plexus now forms a characteristic band across the head. The nose is stubby and the eye is heavily pigmented. (From Nishimura, H., et al.: Prenatal Development of the Human with Special Reference to Craniofacial Structures: An Atlas. Washington, DC, National Institutes of Health, 1977.)

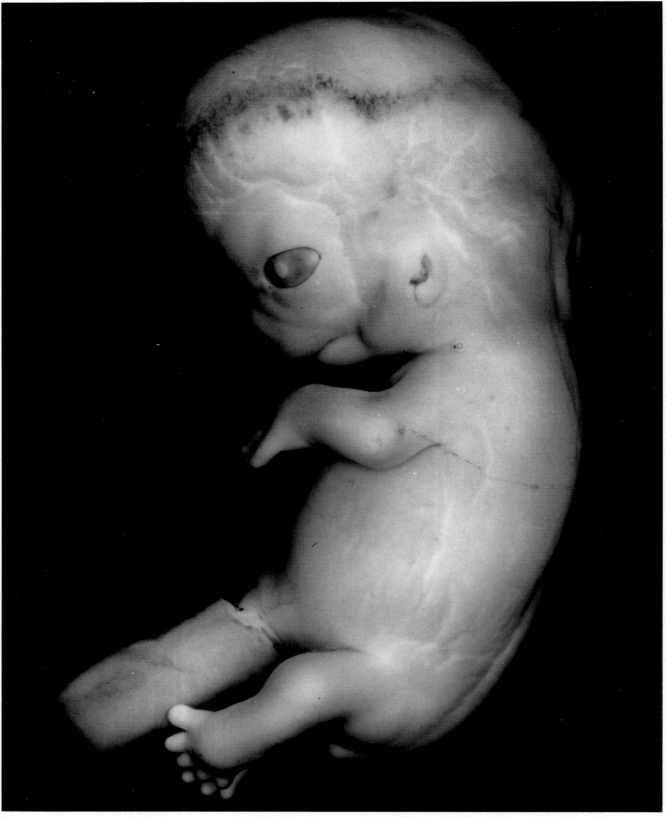

A

Figure 2–24. *See legend on the following page.*

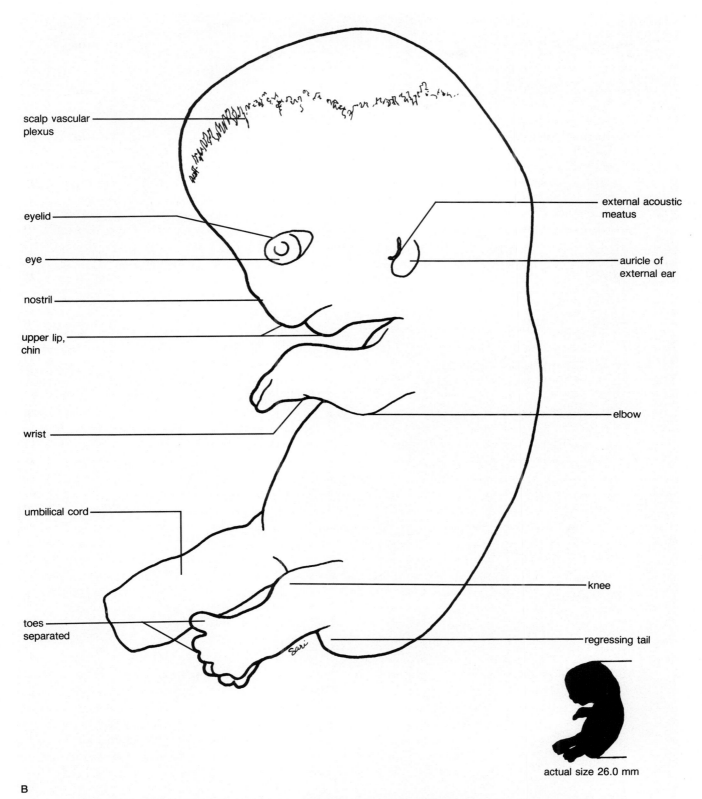

scalp vascular
plexus

eyelid

eye

nostril

upper lip,
chin

wrist

umbilical cord

toes
separated

external acoustic
meatus

auricle of
external ear

elbow

knee

regressing tail

actual size 26.0 mm

B

Figure 2–24. *A,* Lateral view of an embryo at Carnegie stage 22, about 54 days. *B,* Drawing indicating the structures shown in *A.* The toes are separate but short. The eyelids and auricle are well developed. The chin and jaw are distinctive but underdeveloped due to the absence of teeth. The tail has almost disappeared. (From Nishimura, H., et al.: Prenatal Development of the Human with Special Reference to Craniofacial Structures: An Atlas. Washington, DC, National Institutes of Health, 1977.)

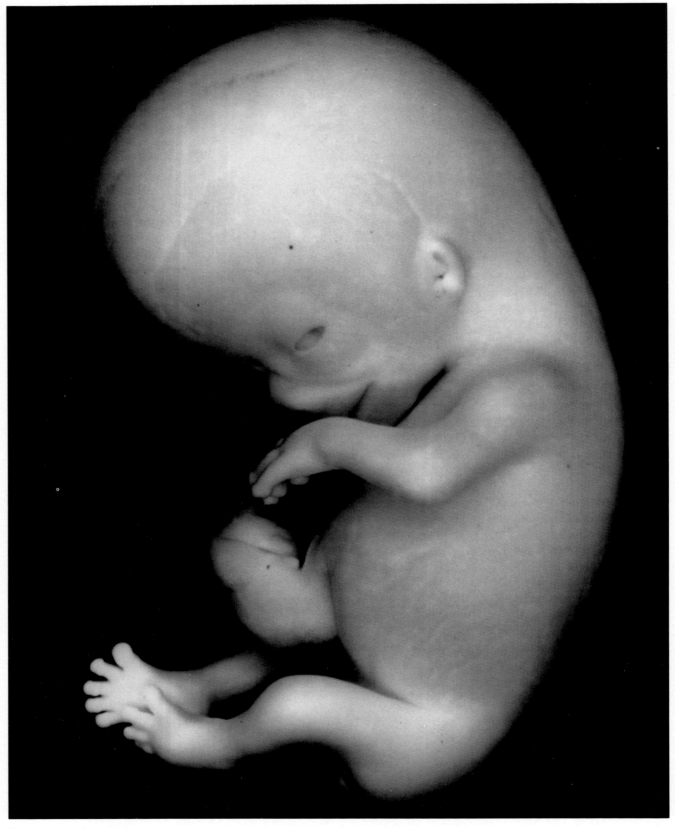

A

Figure 2–25.   *See legend on the following page.*

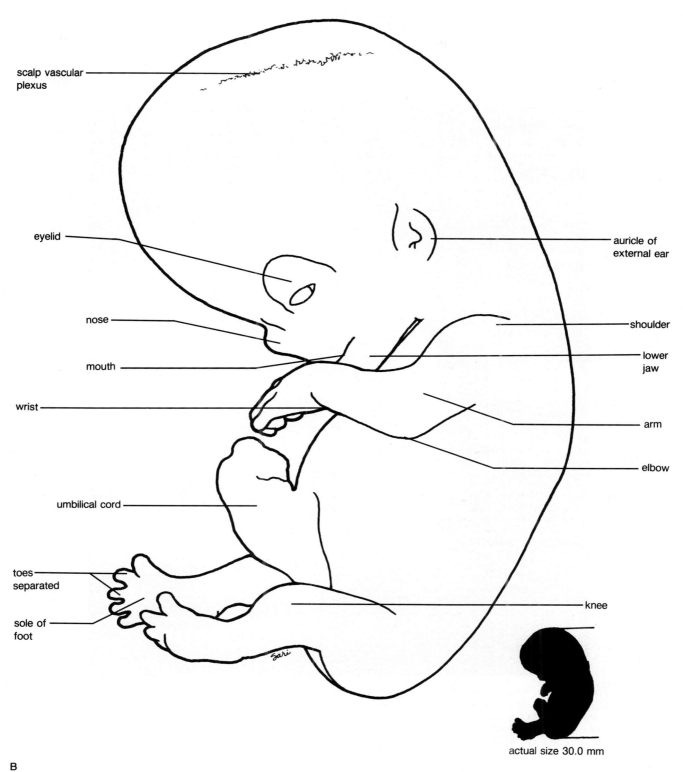

scalp vascular
plexus

eyelid

nose

mouth

wrist

umbilical cord

toes
separated

sole of
foot

auricle of
external ear

shoulder

lower
jaw

arm

elbow

knee

actual size 30.0 mm

B

Figure 2–25. *A,* Lateral view of an embryo at Carnegie stage 23, about 56 days (see also Fig. 2–26). *B,* Drawing indicating the structures shown in *A.* The eyelids are closer to each other (compare with Fig. 2–24). The scalp vascular plexus is reduced and the tail has disappeared. The embryo now has a distinct human appearance. (From Nishimura, H., et al.: Prenatal Development of the Human with Special Reference to Craniofacial Structures: An Atlas. Washington, DC, National Institutes of Health, 1977.)

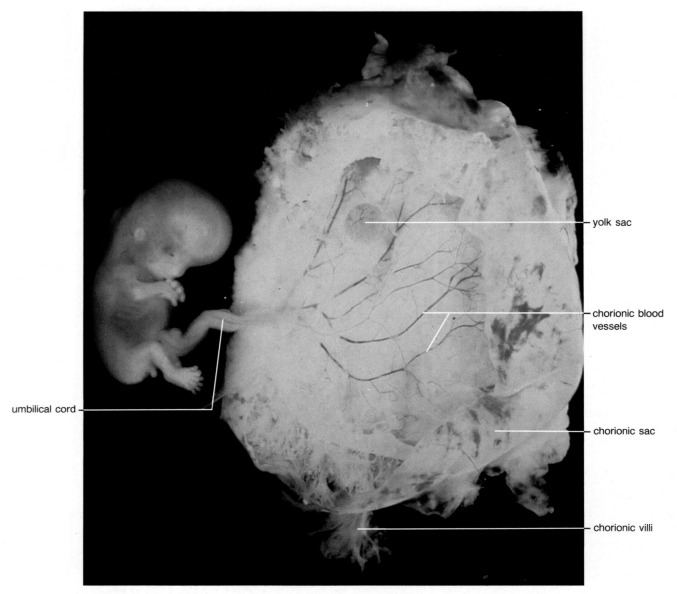

Figure 2-26. Photograph of an embryo at Carnegie stage 23, about 56 days. The embryo has been removed from its chorionic sac. The yolk sac is very small at this stage and will soon disappear (compare with Fig. 4-3A). Note the large size of the head in comparison to the rest of the body. Although the phallus is large, sex cannot be determined externally at this stage because the primordial genital organ is similar in both sexes at this age (see Chapter 10).

TABLE 2-1. CRITERIA FOR ESTIMATING DEVELOPMENTAL STAGES IN HUMAN EMBRYOS

Age (Days)	Figure Reference	Carnegie Stage	No. of Somites	Length (mm)*	Main External Characteristics†
20–21	2–7	9	1–3	1.5–3.0	*Flat embryonic disc. Deep neural groove and prominent neural folds.* One to three pairs of somites present. Head fold evident.
22–23	2–8	10	4–12	2.0–3.5	*Embryo straight or slightly curved. Neural tube forming or formed opposite somites,* but widely open at rostral and caudal neuropores. First and second pairs of branchial arches visible.
24–25	2–9	11	13–20	2.5–4.5	*Embryo curved owing to head and tail folds.* Rostral neuropore closing. Otic placodes present. Optic vesicles formed.
26–27	2–10	12	21–29	3.0–5.0	*Upper limb buds appear.* Rostral neuropore closed. Caudal neuropore closing. Three pairs of branchial arches visible. Heart prominence distinct. Otic pits present.
28–30	2–11	13	30–35	4.0–6.0	*Embryo has C-shaped curve.* Caudal neuropore closed. Upper limb buds are flipper-like. Four pairs of branchial arches visible. *Lower limb buds appear. Otic vesicles present.* Lens placodes distinct. Attenuated *tail* present.
31–32	2–15	14	‡	5.0–7.0	*Upper limbs are paddle-shaped.* Lens pits and nasal pits visible. Optic cups present.
33–36	2–16	15		7.0–9.0	*Hand plates formed; digital rays present.* Lens visicles present. Nasal pits prominent. *Lower limbs are paddle-shaped.* Cervical sinuses visible.
37–40	2–17	16		8.0–11.0	*Foot plates formed.* Pigment visible in retina. Auricular hillocks developing.
41–43	2–19	17		11.0–14.0	*Digital rays clearly visible in hand plates.* Auricular hillocks outline future auricle of external ear. Trunk beginning to straighten. Cerebral vesicles prominent.
44–46	2–20	18		13.0–17.0	*Digital rays clearly visible in foot plates.* Elbow region visible. Eyelids forming. Notches between the digital rays in the hands. Nipples visible.
47–48	2–21	19		16.0–18.0	*Limbs extend ventrally.* Trunk elongating and straightening. Midgut herniation prominent.
49–51	2–22	20		18.0–22.0	*Upper limbs longer and bent at elbows. Fingers distinct but webbed.* Notches between the digital rays in the feet. Scalp vascular plexus appears.
52–53	2–23	21		22.0–24.0	*Hands and feet approach each other. Fingers are free and longer. Toes distinct but webbed.* Stubby tail present.
54–55	2–24	22		23.0–28.0	*Toes free and longer.* Eyelids and auricles of external ears more developed.
56	2–25 2–26	23		27.0–31.0	*Head more rounded and shows human characteristics.* External genitalia still have sexless appearance. Distinct bulge still present in umbilical cord, caused by herniation of intestines. *Tail has disappeared.*

* The embryonic lengths indicate the usual range, but they do not indicate the full range within a given stage, especially when specimens of poor quality are included. In stages 10 and 11, the measurement is greatest length *(GL);* in subsequent stages crown-rump *(CR)* measurements are given.
† Based on Nishimura et al. (1974), O'Rahilly and Müller (1987, 1992), and Shiota (1991).
‡ At this and subsequent stages, the number of somites is difficult to determine and so is not a useful criterion.
(From Moore KL, Persaud TVN; *The Developing Human,* ed 5. Philadelphia, W B Saunders, 1993.)

3
THE NINTH TO THIRTY-EIGHTH WEEKS OF HUMAN DEVELOPMENT

Development during the **fetal period** (ninth to thirty-eighth weeks) is primarily concerned with rapid growth of the body and differentiation of tissues and organs that started to develop during the embryonic period (see Chapter 2). A notable change occurring during the fetal period is the relative slowdown in the growth of the head compared with the rest of the body. The rate of body growth during the fetal period is rapid, especially between the ninth and sixteenth weeks (Fig. 3–1), and fetal weight gain is phenomenal during the terminal weeks.

ESTIMATION OF FETAL AGE

If doubt arises about the age of a fetus, sonographic measurements are taken to determine its size and probable age, and to provide a reliable prediction of the *expected date of confinement* (EDC) for delivery of the fetus. The intrauterine period may be divided into days, weeks, or months, but confusion arises if it is not stated whether the age is calculated from: (1) the onset of the last normal menstrual period (LNMP), or (2) the estimated day of fertilization (see Fig. 1–1). Most uncertainty arises when months are used, particularly when it is not stated whether calendar months (28 to 31 days) or lunar months (28 days) are meant. Fetal age in this atlas is calculated from the estimated time of fertilization, and months refer to calendar months. It is best to express fetal age in weeks and to state whether the beginning or end of a week is meant because statements such as "in the tenth week" are nonspecific.

Various measurements and external characteristics are useful for estimating fetal age. *Crown rump length* (CRL) is usually the most reliable measurement, but the length of fetuses, like that of infants, varies considerably for a given age. Foot length correlates well with CRL and is particularly useful for estimating the age of incomplete or macerated fetuses. *Fetal weight* is often a useful criterion for estimating age, but there may be a discrepancy between the fertilization age and the weight of a fetus, particularly when the mother has had metabolic disturbances during pregnancy, e.g., diabetes mellitus. In these cases, fetal weight often exceeds values considered normal for CRL.

Fetal dimensions obtained from ultrasound measurements of fetuses closely approximate CRL measurements obtained from aborted fetuses. *Ultrasound CRL measurements* are now predictive of fetal age with an accuracy of ± one to two days (Fig. 3–2). In addition, the biparietal diameter of the head and the dimension of the trunk may be obtained. At 9 weeks, the head is still slightly larger than the trunk.

The Fetal Period

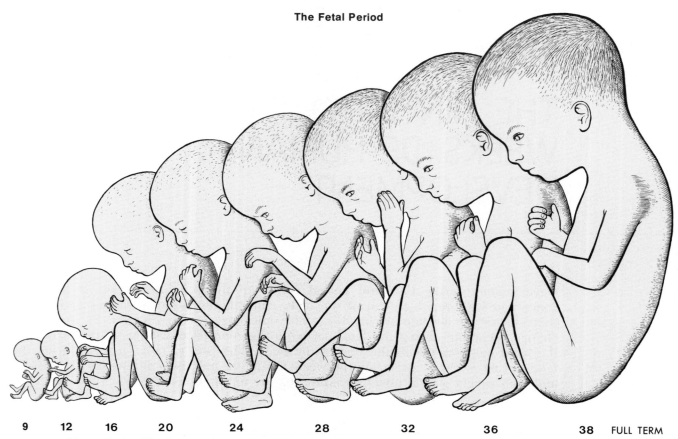

| 9 | 12 | 16 | 20 | 24 | 28 | 32 | 36 | 38 | FULL TERM |

Figure 3–1. The fetal period, extending from the ninth week to birth, is characterized by growth and elaboration of tissues and organs. Sex is clearly distinguishable by 12 weeks. Fetuses become viable at 22 weeks, but their chances of survival are not good until they are several weeks older. In this drawing, 9- to 38-week fetuses are shown at about half their actual size. Note that head hair begins to appear at 20 weeks, and that eyebrows and eyelashes are recognizable by 24 weeks. Observe that the eyelids are fused at 9 weeks and open at 26 weeks.

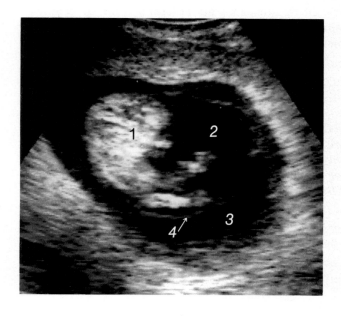

Figure 3–2. Transvaginal ultrasound scan of a fetus (1) early in the ninth week, showing its relationship to the amniotic cavity (2), the extrafetal or chorionic cavity (3), and amnion (4). (From Wathen NC, Cass PL, Kitan MJ, Chard T: *Prenatal Diagnosis 11*:145, 1991. Reprinted by permission of John Wiley & Sons, Ltd.).

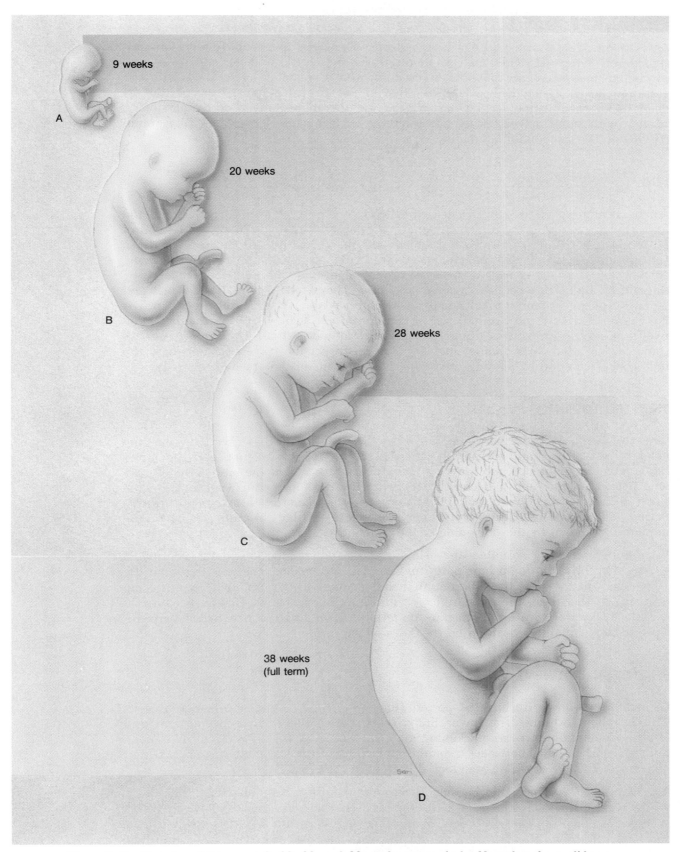

Figure 3–3. Drawing of fetuses at 9, 20, 28, and 38 weeks, respectively. Note that the eyelids are fused in 9- and 20-week fetuses. They are usually open at 26 weeks. During the last two months, the fetus obtains well-rounded contours due to the deposition of subcutaneous fat.

Assessment of fetal size and age is enhanced when head and trunk dimensions are considered along with CRL measurements. Recently, cheek-to-cheek and transverse cerebellar measurements have been used for the assessment of fetal growth and gestational age, respectively. Determination of the size of a fetus, especially of its head, is of great value to the obstetrician for the management of patients, e.g., women with small pelves and/or those fetuses with intrauterine growth retardation (IUGR) and/or congenital anomalies.

NINE TO TWELVE WEEKS

At the beginning of the ninth week, the head constitutes one half the CRL of the fetus. Subsequently, growth in body length accelerates rapidly so that, by the end of 12 weeks, the CRL has more than doubled. Although growth of the head slows down considerably, it is still disproportionately large compared with the rest of the body. At 9 weeks the face is broad, the eyes widely separated, the ears low-set, and, by the end of the ninth week, *the eyelids are fused.* The external genitalia of males and females appear similar until the end of the ninth week. Their mature fetal form is not established until the twelfth week. *Urine formation* begins between the ninth and twelfth weeks, and urine is discharged into the amniotic fluid. The fetus reabsorbs some of this fluid after swallowing it. Fetal waste products are transferred to the maternal circulation by passing across the placental membrane (see Chapter 4).

THIRTEEN TO SIXTEEN WEEKS

Growth is very rapid during this period (Figs. 3–1, 3–3, and 3–4). By 16 weeks, the head is relatively small compared with that of the 12-week fetus, and the lower limbs have lengthened. Limb movements, which first occur at the end of the embryonic period (eight weeks), become coordinated by the fourteenth week but are too slight to be felt by the mother. *Ossification of the skeleton* is active during this period (see Fig. 12–4), and the bones are clearly visible on radiographs of the mother's abdomen by the beginning of the sixteenth week.

Ultrasonography has revealed that slow *eye movements occur at 14 weeks* (16 weeks after LNMP). Scalp hair patterning is also determined during this period. By 16 weeks, the ovaries are differentiated and contain primordial follicles enclosing oogonia. At this time, the appearance of the fetus is even more human because its eyes face anteriorly rather than anterolaterally. In addition, the external ears are close to their definitive position on the sides of the head.

SEVENTEEN TO TWENTY WEEKS

Growth slows down during this period (Fig. 3–1), but the fetus still increases its CRL by about 50 mm. The lower limbs reach their final relative proportions and fetal movements known as **quickening** are commonly felt by the mother. The mean time that intervenes between a mother's first detection of fetal movements and delivery is 147 days, with a standard deviation of ±15 days.

The skin at 17 weeks is thin because there is very little subcutaneous fat (Fig. 3–5). By 18 weeks, the skin is covered with a greasy, cheeselike material known as *vernix caseosa.* It consists of a mixture of dead epidermal cells and a fatty secretion from the fetal sebaceous glands of the skin. The vernix caseosa protects the delicate fetal skin from abrasions, chapping, and hardening that could result from its exposure to amniotic fluid. The bodies of 20-week fetuses are usually completely covered with fine downy hair called *lanugo;* this hair helps to hold the vernix caseosa on the skin. Eyebrows and head hair are also visible at 20 weeks (Fig. 3–3).

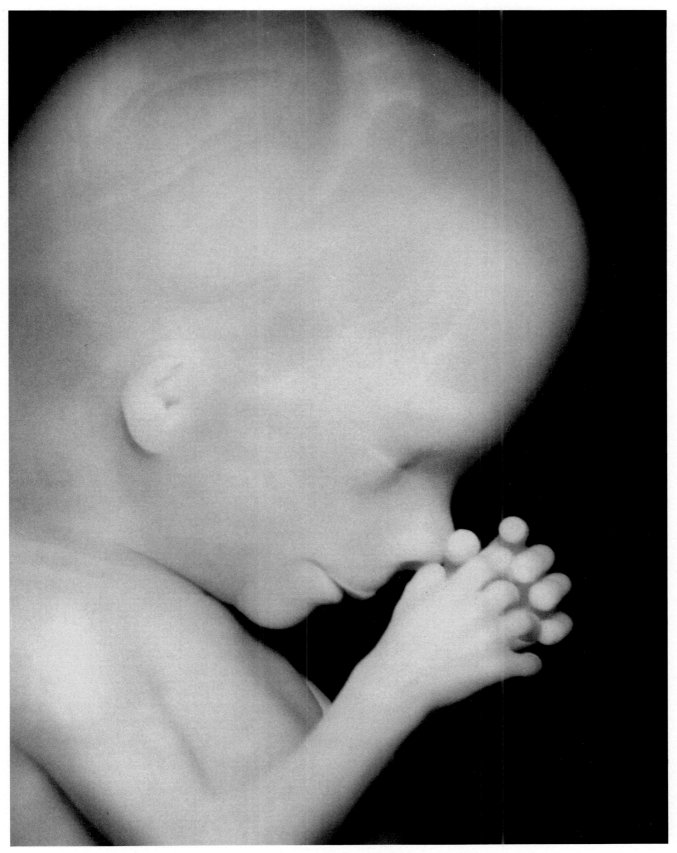

Figure 3–4. Enlarged photograph of a 13-week fetus. The crown-rump length is 84 mm. Note that the eyelids are fused and that the ear stands out from the head. A fetus at this stage has no chance of survival outside of the uterus due to the immaturity of the lungs (Courtesy of Professor Jean Hay, Department of Anatomy, Faculty of Medicine, University of Manitoba, Winnipeg, Canada).

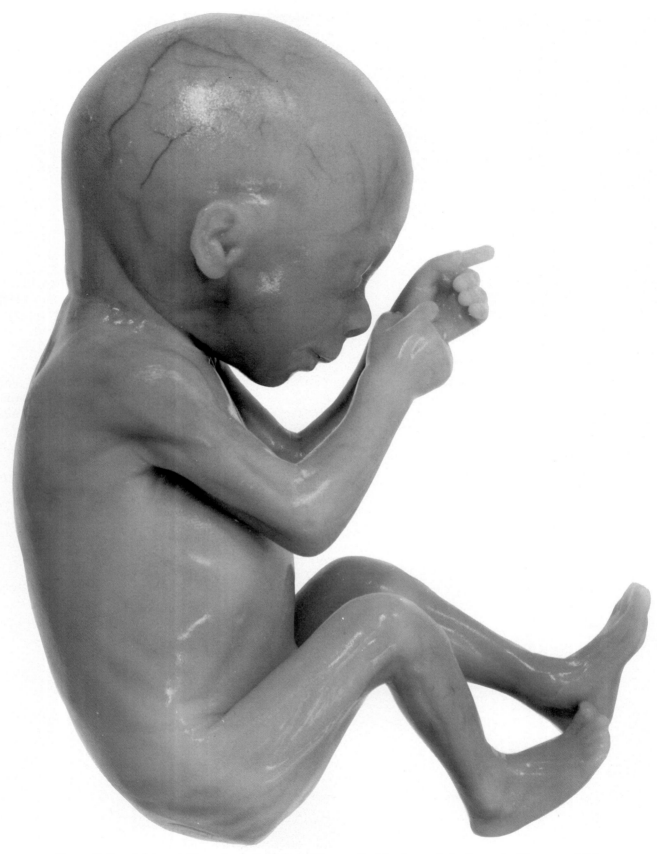

Figure 3–5. A fetus at 17 weeks (actual size). Observe the blood vessels in the scalp. They are visible because the skin is thin at this stage and very little subcutaneous fat is present. Although it appears mature, a fetus at this stage is unable to survive if it aborts spontaneously, as in this case.

Brown fat forms during the seventeenth through twentieth weeks and is the site of heat production, particularly in the neonate. This specialized adipose tissue produces heat by oxidizing fatty acids. Brown fat is chiefly found at the root of the neck, posterior to the sternum, and in the perirenal area (England, 1983). Brown fat has a high content of mitochondria, giving it a definite brown hue.

By 18 weeks, the uterus is formed and canalization of the vagina has begun. By 20 weeks, the *testes* have begun to descend but are still located on the posterior abdominal wall, as are the *ovaries* in female fetuses. By this time many *primordial ovarian follicles* containing oogonia have formed.

TWENTY-ONE TO TWENTY-FIVE WEEKS

There is a *substantial weight gain* during this period. Although still somewhat lean, the fetus is better proportioned (Fig. 3–6). The skin is usually wrinkled, particularly during the early part of this period, and is more translucent. The skin is pink to red in fresh specimens because blood is visible in the capillaries. At 21 weeks, rapid eye movements begin, and *blink-startle responses* have been reported at 22 to 23 weeks following application of a vibroacoustic noise source to the mother's abdomen (Birnholz and Benaceraff, 1983).

By 24 weeks, the secretory epithelial cells (type II pneumocytes) in the interalveolar walls of the lung have begun to secrete *surfactant,* a surface-active lipid that maintains the patency of the developing alveoli of the lungs (see Chapter 8). *Fingernails* are also present by 24 weeks. Although a 22- to 25-week fetus born prematurely may survive if given intensive care, it may die during early infancy because its respiratory system is still immature.

TWENTY-SIX TO TWENTY-NINE WEEKS

During this period, a prematurely born fetus often survives if given intensive care because its *lungs are now capable of breathing air.* The lungs and pulmonary vasculature have developed sufficiently to provide adequate gas exchange (Fig. 3–7). In addition, the central nervous system has matured to the stage where it can direct rhythmic breathing movements and control body temperature. The greatest neonatal losses occur in infants who weigh less than 2000 gm (Bowie, 1988).

The eyes reopen at 26 weeks, and lanugo and head hair are well developed (Fig. 3–6). Toenails become visible, and considerable subcutaneous fat is now present under the skin, smoothing out many of the wrinkles. During this period, the quantity of white fat increases to about 3.5 per cent of body weight. *The fetal spleen is now an important site of hematopoiesis.* Erythropoiesis in the spleen ends by 28 weeks, by which time bone marrow has become the major site of formation of erythrocytes.

THIRTY TO THIRTY-FOUR WEEKS

The *pupillary light reflex* of the eyes can be elicited by 30 weeks. Usually by the end of this period, the skin is pink and smooth, and the upper and lower limbs have a chubby appearance. At this stage the quantity of white fat is about 8 per cent of body weight. Fetuses 32 weeks and older usually survive if born prematurely. If a normal-weight fetus is born during this period, it is "premature by date" as opposed to being "premature by weight."

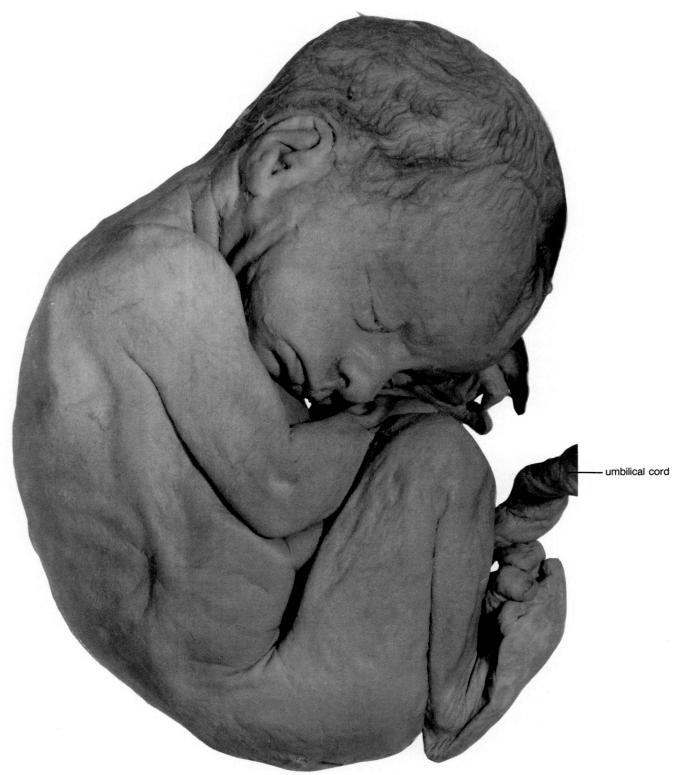

umbilical cord

Figure 3–6. Photograph of a 25-week fetus in the fetal position (actual size). Note that its fingernails are present and that the skin is wrinkled and the body lean due to the scarcity of subcutaneous fat. A fetus born prematurely at this age may survive. Observe that its eyelids are just beginning to separate. They are usually wide open at 26 weeks.

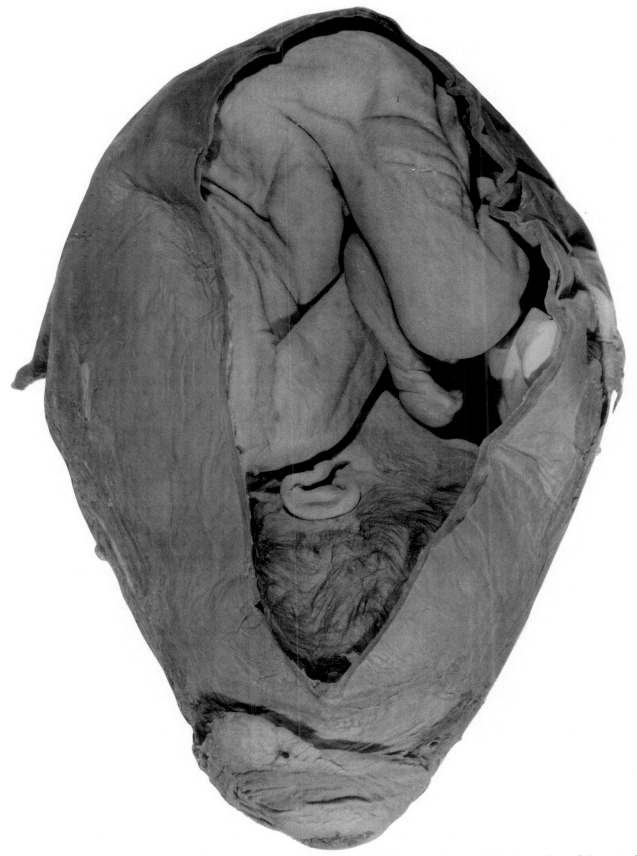

Figure 3–7. Photograph of a 29-week fetus in the cephalic presentation in utero (actual size). A portion of the anterior wall of the uterus and its membranes (amnion and chorion) have been cut away to expose the fetus. At this age the breech (caudal end of fetus) is commonly in the fundus of the uterus and the head is adjacent to the cervix. Fetuses born at this age usually survive because their lungs are capable of breathing air. This fetus and its mother died due to injuries sustained in an automobile accident.

THIRTY-FIVE TO THIRTY-EIGHT WEEKS

Fetuses at 35 weeks have a firm grasp and exhibit a spontaneous orientation to light. As term approaches, the nervous system is sufficiently mature to carry out some integrative functions. Most fetuses during this "finishing period" are plump (Fig. 3–8). By 36 weeks, the circumferences of the head and abdomen are approximately equal. After this, the circumference of the abdomen may be greater than that of the head. There is a *slowing of growth* as the time of birth approaches. Normal fetuses usually reach a CRL of 360 mm and weigh 3200 to 3400 gm. By full term the amount of white fat is about 16 per cent of body weight. A fetus adds about 14 gm of fat a day during these last weeks of gestation. In general, male fetuses are longer and weigh more at birth than females.

By full term (38 weeks after fertilization; 40 weeks after LNMP), the skin is normally bluish-pink. The chest is prominent and the breasts protrude slightly in both sexes. The testes are usually in the scrotum in full-term male infants; their descent begins at 28 to 32 weeks. Thus, premature male infants commonly have undescended testes. Although the head at full term is smaller in relation to the rest of the body than it was earlier in fetal life, it still is one of the largest regions of the fetus. This is an important consideration related to its passage through the birth canal (Fig. 3–12; also see Fig. 4–9).

THE TIME OF BIRTH

The expected time of birth is 266 days or 38 weeks after fertilization, i.e., 280 days or 40 weeks after LNMP. However, about 12 per cent of babies are born one to two weeks after the expected date of confinement (EDC). Prolongation of pregnancy for three or more weeks beyond the EDC occurs in 5 to 6 per cent of women. Some infants in prolonged pregnancies develop the *postmaturity syndrome.* They are thin and have dry, parchmentlike skin, but they are often overweight and characterized by absence of lanugo hair, decreased or absent vernix caseosa, long nails, and increased alertness. When delivery is delayed three weeks or more beyond term, there is a significant increase in mortality. Because of this, labor is often induced.

The common clinical method of determining EDC is to count back three calendar months from the first day of the LNMP and then add a year and seven days *(Naegele's rule).* In women with regular menstrual cycles, this method gives a reasonably accurate EDC. If the woman's cycles were irregular, however, miscalculations of two to three weeks may occur. In addition, *implantation bleeding* occurs in some pregnant women at the time of the first missed period (about two weeks after fertilization [see Fig. 1–5]). Should the woman interpret this bleeding as a normal menstruation, the estimated time of birth could be miscalculated by two or more weeks. Ultrasonographic examinations of the fetus, in particular CRL measurements between 9 and 12 weeks of gestation (7 to 10 weeks after fertilization), are commonly used now for obtaining a more reliable prediction of the EDC (Fig. 3–2).

PERINATOLOGY

This branch of medicine is concerned with the well-being of the fetus and neonate, generally covering the period from about 26 weeks after fertilization to four weeks after birth. The subspecialty of *perinatal medicine* combines certain aspects of obstetrics and pediatrics. A physician can now determine whether or not a fetus has a particular disease or a congenital anomaly by using various diagnostic techniques. *Prenatal diagnosis* can be made early enough to allow early termination of the pregnancy if elected, e.g., when serious anomalies incompatible with postnatal life are diagnosed (e.g., trisomy 13; see Fig. 5–8). In selected cases, various treatments

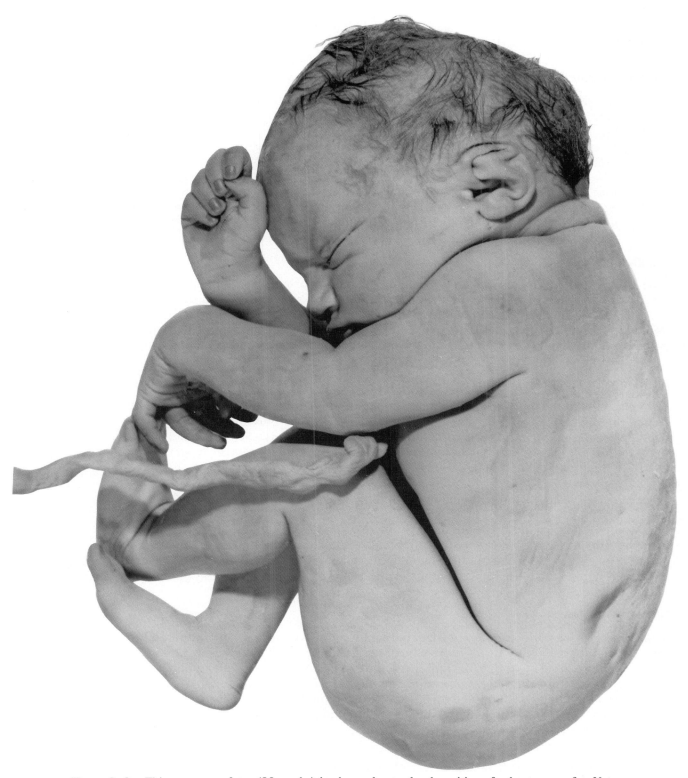

Figure 3–8. This near-term fetus (36 weeks) is plump due to the deposition of subcutaneous fat. Note that its fingernails have reached its fingertips. A fetus born at this age has an excellent chance of survival.

can be given to the fetus, e.g., the administration of drugs to correct cardiac arrhythmia (Harrison, 1991). Surgical correction of some congenital anomalies in utero is also possible, e.g., ureterostomies on fetuses that have ureters that do not open into the bladder.

Chorionic Villus Sampling (CVS)

Biopsies of chorionic villi may be obtained by inserting a needle, guided by ultrasonography, through the mother's abdominal and uterine walls into the uterine cavity (Fig. 3–9A). CVS is commonly performed transcervically using real-time ultrasound guidance (Hogge, 1991). Biopsies of chorionic villi are used for detecting chromosomal abnormalities, inborn errors of metabolism, and X-linked disorders. CVS can be performed as early as the ninth week of gestation (seven weeks after fertilization). The rate of fetal loss is about 1 per cent, slightly more than the risk from amniocentesis. The major advantage of CVS over amniocentesis is that it allows the results of chromosomal analysis to be available several weeks earlier.

Diagnostic Amniocentesis

This is the most common invasive prenatal diagnostic procedure (Fig. 3–9B). Amniocentesis is usually performed during the fourteenth to sixteenth weeks of gestation (12 to 14 weeks after fertilization). The procedure is relatively devoid of risk, especially when the procedure is performed by an experienced physician who is guided by ultrasonography for outlining the position of the fetus and placenta.

Alpha-fetoprotein (AFP) Assay

AFP escapes from the circulation into the amniotic fluid from fetuses with *open neural tube defects* (NTDs), such as spina bifida with myeloschisis or meroanencephaly (see Chapter 13). The term "open" refers to lesions that are not covered with skin. AFP also enters the amniotic fluid from open ventral wall defects (VWDs), such as gastroschisis and omphalocele (see Chapter 9).

Percutaneous Umbilical Cord Blood Sampling (PUBS)

Fetal blood samples may be obtained from the umbilical vessels for chromosome analysis. Ultrasonographic scanning facilitates the procedure by outlining the location of the vessels. PUBS is often used about 20 weeks after LNMP for chromosome analysis when ultrasonographic or other examinations have shown a fetal anomaly.

Ultrasonography

The chorionic (gestational) sac and its contents may be visualized during the embryonic and fetal periods by using ultrasound techniques (Fig. 3–2). Placental and fetal sizes, multiple births, and abnormal presentations can also be determined. *Sonograms* give accurate measurements of the biparietal diameter of the fetal skull from which close estimates of fetal age and length can be made. *Neural tube defects,* such as meroanencephaly (anencephaly) and myelomeningocele, can easily be detected (Figs. 3–10 and 3–11).

Computed Tomography (CT) and Magnetic Resonance Imaging (MRI)

When planning fetal treatment, CT and MRI (Figs. 3–12 and 3–13) may be used to provide more information about an abnormality that has been detected in a sonogram. The major application of CT is in performing *pelvimetry* (measurement of the diameters of the pelvis). The uses of MRI are in the assessment of the cervix, uterus, and placenta, and in the investigation of certain fetal anomalies.

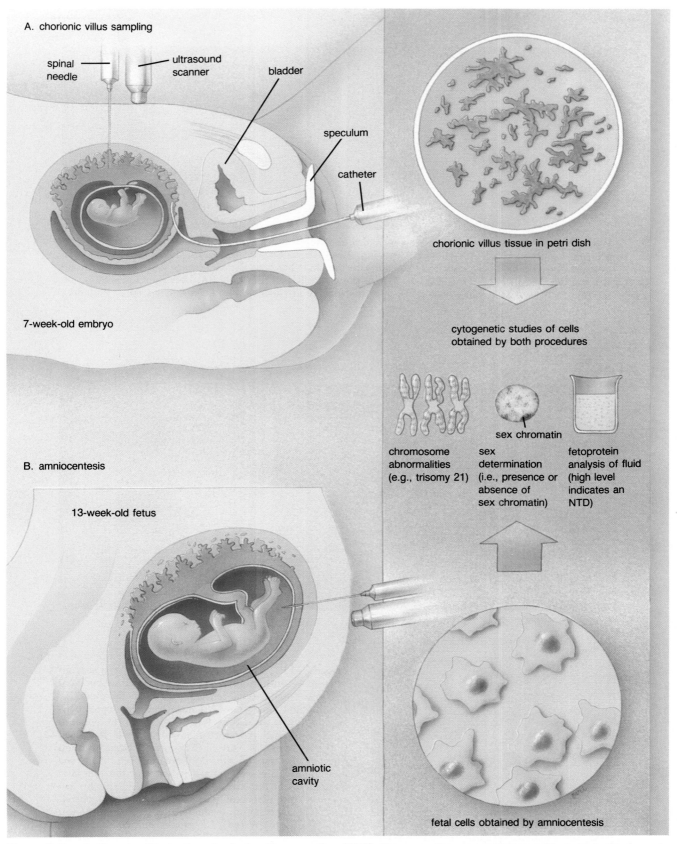

A. chorionic villus sampling

spinal needle

ultrasound scanner

bladder

speculum

catheter

chorionic villus tissue in petri dish

7-week-old embryo

cytogenetic studies of cells obtained by both procedures

sex chromatin

B. amniocentesis

chromosome abnormalities (e.g., trisomy 21)

sex determination (i.e., presence or absence of sex chromatin)

fetoprotein analysis of fluid (high level indicates an NTD)

13-week-old fetus

amniotic cavity

fetal cells obtained by amniocentesis

Figure 3–9. *A*, Drawing illustrating chorionic villus sampling (CVS). Two sampling approaches are illustrated: (1) through the maternal anterior abdominal wall with a spinal needle, and (2) by way of the vagina and cervical canal using a malleable cannula. Success and safety in this approach depend upon use of a ultrasound scanner. CVS can be performed as early as the ninth week of gestation (seven weeks after fertilization). *B*, Drawing illustrating amniocentesis. A needle is inserted through the abdominal and uterine walls into the amniotic cavity. A syringe is attached and amniotic fluid is withdrawn for diagnostic purposes (e.g., for cell cultures). Before the procedure is carried out, the placenta is located by ultrasonography so it can be avoided when the needle is inserted. The technique is usually performed at 14 to 15 weeks of gestation (12 to 13 weeks after fertilization). Prior to this stage of development, there is relatively little amniotic fluid and the difficulties in obtaining it without endangering the mother or fetus are consequently greater.

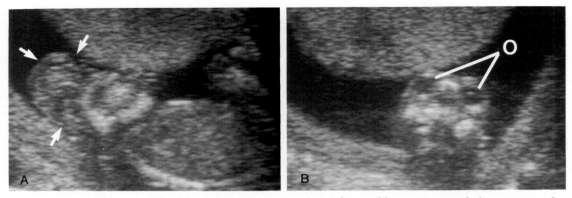

Figure 3–10. Early second trimester pregnancy showing a fetus with meroanencephaly or anencephaly (partial absence of the brain [see also Fig. 13–12]). *A,* Sagittal sonogram demonstrating a large mass of angiomatous tissue *(arrows)* cephalad to the skull base. *B,* Coronal image of the face demonstrating the absence of the calvaria superior to the orbits (O). (From Filly RA: Ultrasound evaluation of the fetal neural axis. In Callen PW (ed): *Ultrasonography in Obstetrics and Gynecology,* ed 2. Philadelphia, WB Saunders, 1988.)

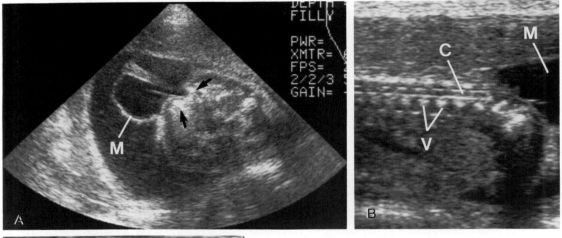

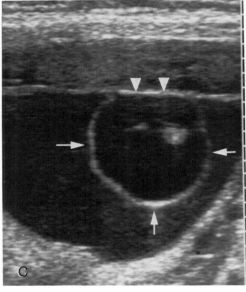

Figure 3–11. *A,* Transverse sonogram of the sacrum in a fetus with a myelomeningocele (M). Abnormal posterior ossification centers are seen *(arrows)*. *B,* Longitudinal sonogram demonstrating the myelomeningocele (M) extending from the vertebral column. The spinal cord (C) ends at an abnormally low level (tethered cord). V, vertebral bodies. *C,* Scan oriented through the sac of the myelomeningocele. The sac margin is easily seen where it contacts the amniotic fluid *(arrows)* but virtually disappears where the sac contacts the placental surface *(arrowheads)*. (From Filly RA: Ultrasound evaluation of the fetal neural axis. *In* Callen PW (ed): *Ultrasonography in Obstetrics and Gynecology,* ed 2. Philadelphia, WB Saunders, 1988.)

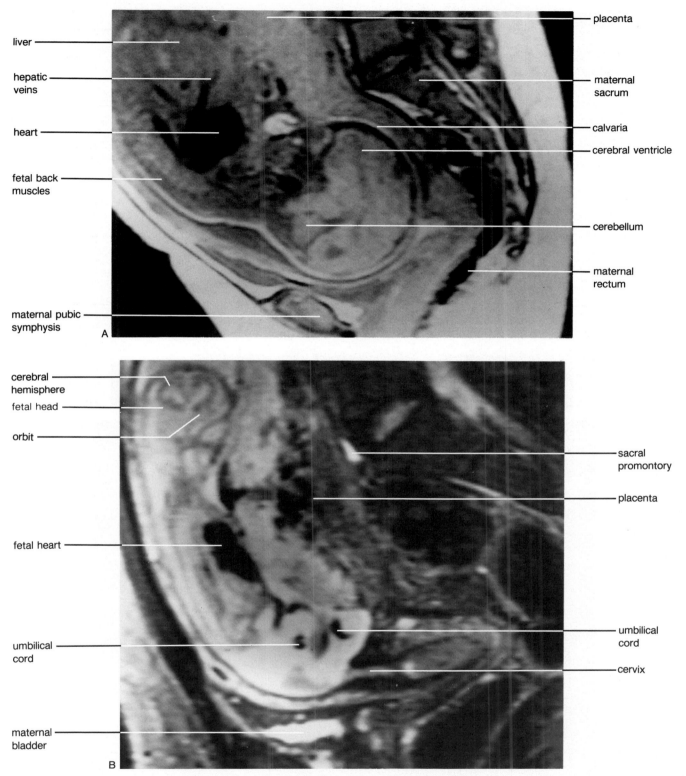

liver

hepatic veins

heart

fetal back muscles

maternal pubic symphysis

A

placenta

maternal sacrum

calvaria

cerebral ventricle

cerebellum

maternal rectum

cerebral hemisphere

fetal head

orbit

fetal heart

umbilical cord

maternal bladder

B

sacral promontory

placenta

umbilical cord

cervix

Figure 3–12. Sagittal magnetic resonance images (MRIs) of the pelves of pregnant women. *A,* The fetus is in the cephalic presentation. The brain, heart, liver, and hepatic veins are well shown, as is the placenta. *B,* The fetus, placenta, and umbilical cord are visible. Note the ventricles of the cerebrum. (Courtesy of Dr. Shirley McCarthy, Director of MRI, Department of Diagnostic Radiology, Yale University School of Medicine, New Haven, Connecticut.)

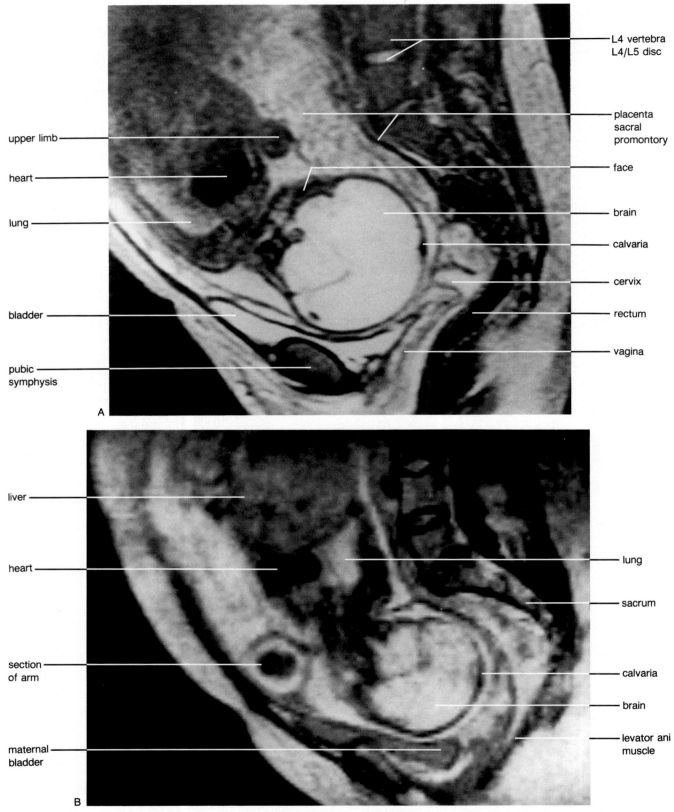

Figure 3–13.   Sagittal magnetic resonance (MR) scans through the pelves of pregnant women. *A,* The fetal head is juxtaposed to the cervix. *B,* The fetal head is opposite the maternal sacrum. Note the heart, lung, arm, placenta, and umbilical cord. (Courtesy of Dr. Shirley McCarthy, Director of MRI, Department of Diagnostic Radiology, Yale University School of Medicine, New Haven, Connecticut.)

4

PLACENTA AND FETAL MEMBRANES

The placenta is a **fetomaternal organ** that has two components: (1) a *fetal portion* that develops from the chorionic sac, and (2) a *maternal portion* that is derived from the endometrium (Fig. 4–1). The placenta and umbilical cord function as a *transport mechanism* between the mother and the fetus. Oxygen and nutrients pass from the maternal blood through the placenta to the fetus for its nourishment, and carbon dioxide and waste materials pass from the fetus to the mother for disposal.

The fetal membranes and placenta perform the following functions and activities: protection, nutrition, respiration, excretion, and hormone production. At birth, the placenta and fetal membranes are expelled from the uterus, which is referred to as the "afterbirth" by lay persons (Fig. 4–9*H*).

The chorion, amnion, yolk sac, and allantois constitute the fetal membranes, which develop from the zygote but do not form parts of the embryo or fetus except for parts of the yolk sac and allantois. Part of the yolk sac is incorporated into the embryo as the primordium of the primitive gut (see Chapter 9). The allantois forms a fibrous cord that is known as the urachus in the fetus and the median umbilical ligament in the adult (see Fig. 10–19). It extends from the apex of the urinary bladder to the umbilicus.

THE DECIDUA

The term decidua (L. *deciduus,* a falling off) is applied to the *gravid endometrium* (the functional layer of the endometrium in a pregnant woman). The name indicates that this part of the endometrium separates ("falls away") from the uterus at *parturition* (childbirth).

Three regions of the decidua are named according to their relation to the implantation site (Fig. 4–1): (1) The part deep to the conceptus that forms the maternal component of the placenta is called the *decidua basalis;* (2) the superficial portion overlying the conceptus is known as the *decidua capsularis;* and (3) all the remaining endometrium is referred to as the *decidua parietalis* (vera). These decidual regions, clearly recognizable during *ultrasonography,* are important in diagnosing early pregnancy (Filly, 1988; Lyons and Levi, 1991).

Up to the eighth week, chorionic villi cover the entire chorionic sac (Figs. 4–1*A* and 4–3). As this sac grows, the villi associated with the decidua capsularis are compressed and the blood supply to them is reduced. These villi soon degenerate, producing a bare area (Figs. 4–1*B* and 4–2*D*) known as the *smooth chorion* or chorion laeve (L. *levis,* smooth). As these villi disappear, those associated with the decidua basalis rapidly increase in number, branch profusely, and enlarge.

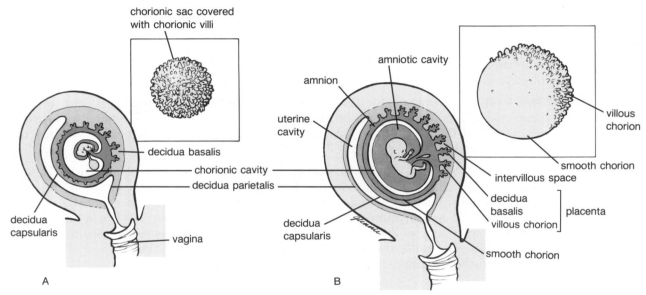

Figure 4-1.   Drawings of sagittal sections of pregnant uteri. *A*, Five weeks. Note that the chorionic sac is completely covered with chorionic villi. *B*, Eight weeks. The chorionic villi have degenerated except where the placenta is forming. The part of the sac lacking villi forms the smooth chorion (see also Fig. 4-8). The villous chorion forms the fetal part of the placenta and the decidua basalis forms its maternal part. (From Moore KL, Persaud TVN: The Developing Human, ed 5. Philadelphia, WB Saunders, 1993.)

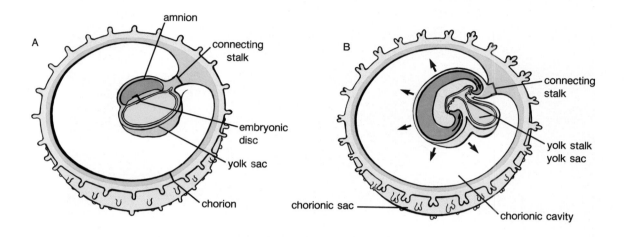

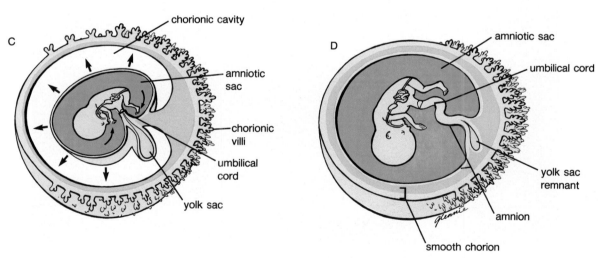

Figure 4–2. Drawings showing how the amnion enlarges, filling the chorionic cavity and ensheathing the umbilical cord to form its epithelial covering. Observe that part of the yolk sac is incorporated into the embryo as the primordial gut. The remnant of the yolk sac is attached to the gut by a narrow yolk stalk. *A,* Three weeks. *B,* Four weeks. *C,* Ten weeks. *D,* 20 weeks. The yolk sac degenerates and is not usually visible after this time. (From Moore KL, Persaud TVN: The Developing Human, ed 5. Philadelphia, WB Saunders, 1993.)

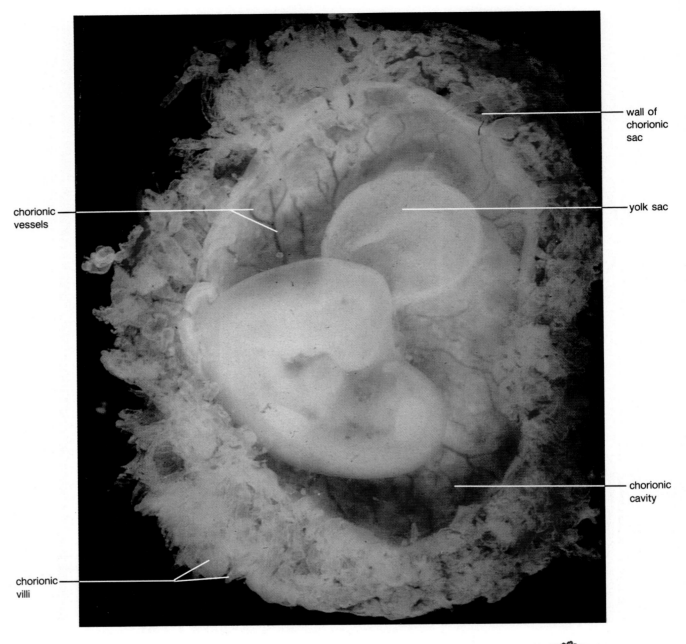

wall of
chorionic
sac

chorionic
vessels

yolk sac

chorionic
cavity

chorionic
villi

actual size of
embryo & its
membranes

A

Figure 4-3. *A,* Lateral view of an embryo at Carnegie stage 14, about 32 days. The chorionic and amniotic sacs have been opened to show the embryo. Note the large size of the yolk sac at this stage (see Fig. 2-15 for the characteristics of an embryo at this stage). The sketch *(lower right)* is drawn to show the actual size of the embryo and its membranes.

Legend continues on the following page.

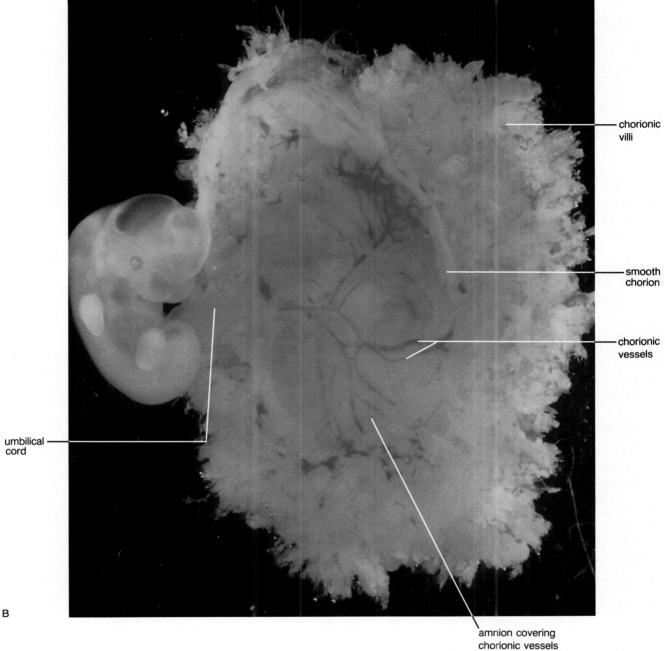

chorionic
villi

smooth
chorion

chorionic
vessels

umbilical
cord

amnion covering
chorionic vessels

B

Figure 4–3. *Continued. B,* Lateral view of an embryo at Carnegie stage 15, about 36 days (see Fig. 2–16 for the characteristics of this embryo). Chorionic villi cover the entire chorionic sac at this stage. (From Nishimura, H., et al.: Prenatal Development of the Human with Special Reference to Craniofacial Structures: An Atlas. Washington, DC, National Institutes of Health, 1977.)

The bushy part of the chorionic sac is known as the *villous chorion* (Fig. 4–1*B*) or chorion frondosum (L. *frondosus,* leafy). The increase in the thickness of the placenta results from the branching of stem villi (Figs. 4–2 to 4–6). As the fetus grows, the uterus and placenta enlarge. Growth in the thickness of the placenta continues until the fetus is about 18 weeks old (20 weeks gestation). The fully developed placenta represents 15 to 30 per cent of the decidua.

The **fetal component of the placenta** is formed by the *villous chorion* (Figs. 4–1, 4–4 to 4–6, and 4–8). The villi project into the intervillous space containing maternal blood. The **maternal component of the placenta** is formed by the *decidua basalis.* This is the endometrium that is related to the fetal component of the placenta (Fig. 4–1). By the end of the fourth month the decidua basalis is largely replaced by the fetal component of the placenta.

The Fetomaternal Junction

The fetal portion of the placenta (villous chorion) is attached to the maternal portion of the placenta (decidua basalis) by the *cytotrophoblastic shell* (Fig. 4–5). Stem chorionic villi ("anchoring villi") are attached firmly to the decidua basalis through the cytotrophoblastic shell. These villi anchor the placenta and fetal membranes to the decidua basalis. Maternal arteries and veins pass freely through gaps in the cytotrophoblastic shell and open into the intervillous space (Figs. 4–4 and 4–5).

PLACENTAL CIRCULATION

The many branch villi of the placenta provide a large surface area where materials are exchanged across the *placental membrane* (barrier) interposed between the fetal and maternal circulations (Figs. 4–4 to 4–7). It is through the numerous *branch villi* which arise from the *stem villi* that the main exchange of material between the mother and fetus takes place. The circulations of the fetus and the mother are separated by the very thin placental membrane consisting of extrafetal tissues (Figs. 4–6 and 4–7).

Fetal Placental Circulation

Poorly oxygenated blood leaves the fetus and passes through the *umbilical arteries* to the placenta. At the site of attachment of the cord to the placenta, these arteries divide into a number of radially disposed vessels that branch freely in the *chorionic plate* before entering the villi (Figs. 4–4 to 4–6). The blood vessels form an extensive *arterio-capillary-venous system* within the villi, which brings the fetal blood extremely close to the maternal blood (Fig. 4–6). This system provides a very large area for the exchange of metabolic and gaseous products between the maternal and fetal blood streams. There is normally *no intermingling of fetal and maternal blood,* but very small amounts of fetal blood may enter the maternal circulation through minute defects that sometimes develop in the placental membrane. The well oxygenated fetal blood passes into thin-walled chorionic veins that follow the chorionic arteries to the site of attachment of the umbilical cord, where they converge to form the *umbilical vein.* This large vessel carries the oxygen-rich blood to the fetus (Figs. 4–4 to 4–6). The fetal circulation is illustrated and discussed in Chapter 11.

Maternal Placental Circulation

The blood in the *intervillous space* is temporarily outside the maternal circulatory system (Figs. 4–5 and 4–6). It enters the intervillous space through 80 to 100 *spiral arteries* in the decidua basalis. These vessels discharge oxygen-rich blood into the intervillous space through gaps in the cytotrophoblastic shell. The blood flow from the spiral arteries is pulsatile and is propelled in jet-like fountains by the maternal

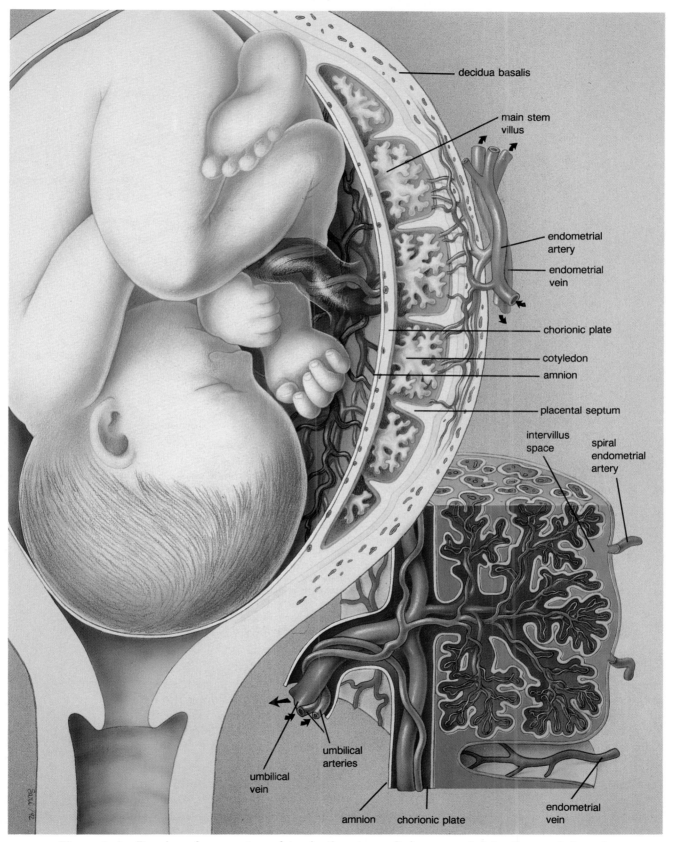

Figure 4–4. Drawing of a near-term fetus in the uterus. It is surrounded by the amniotic and chorionic sacs which have almost obliterated the uterine cavity.

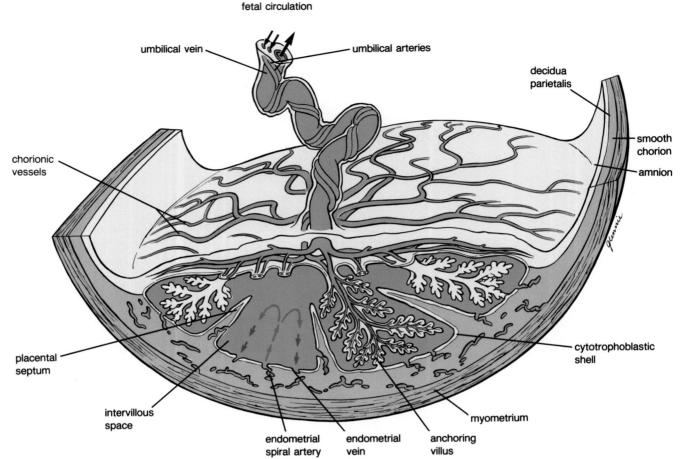

Figure 4–5. Schematic drawing of a section through a mature placenta, showing (1) the relation of the villous chorion (fetal part of placenta) to the decidua basalis (maternal part of placenta), (2) the fetal placental circulation, and (3) the maternal placental circulation. Maternal blood flows into the intervillous space in funnel-shaped spurts from the spiral arteries in the endometrium, and exchanges occur with the fetal blood as the maternal blood flows around the villi. The inflowing arterial blood pushes venous blood out of the intervillous space into the endometrial veins, which are scattered over the entire surface of the decidua basalis. Note that the umbilical arteries carry poorly oxygenated fetal blood (shown in blue) to the placenta, and that the umbilical vein carries well oxygenated blood (shown in red) to the fetus. Note that the cotyledons are separated from each other by placental septa of the maternal portion of the placenta. Each cotyledon consists of two or more main stem villi and their many branches. In this drawing only one main stem villus is shown in each cotyledon, but the stumps of those that have been removed are indicated. See Figure 11–10 for a drawing of the fetal circulation and its relationship to the placenta. (Modified from Moore KL, Persaud TVN: The Developing Human, ed 5. Philadelphia, WB Saunders, 1993.)

blood pressure. The entering blood is at a considerably higher pressure than that in the intervillous space; hence it spurts toward the *chorionic plate* forming the "roof" of the intervillous space. As the pressure dissipates, the blood flows slowly around the branch villi, allowing an exchange of metabolic and gaseous products with the fetal blood. The blood eventually returns to the endometrial veins and the maternal circulation.

The welfare of the embryo and fetus depends more on the adequate bathing of the branch villi with maternal blood than on any other factor. Reductions of uteroplacental circulation (e.g., due to the effects of nicotine in cigarettes) result in fetal hypoxia and IUGR. Severe reductions of uteroplacental circulation can result in fetal death. The intervillous space of the mature placenta contains about 150 ml of blood that is replenished three or four times per minute. The intermittent contractions of

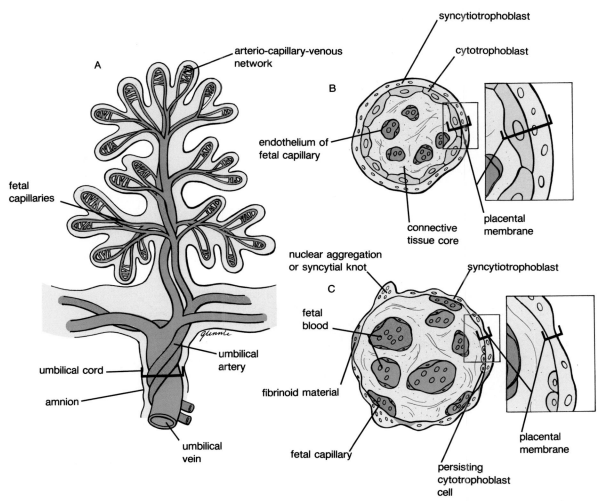

Figure 4–6. *A*, Drawing of a chorionic villus showing its arterio-capillary-venous system carrying fetal blood. The artery carries poorly oxygenated blood and waste products from the fetus, whereas the vein carries well oxygenated blood and nutrients to the fetus. *B* and *C*, Drawings of sections through a chorionic villus at 10 weeks and at full term, respectively. The villi are bathed externally in maternal blood. The placental membrane, composed of extrafetal tissues, separates the maternal blood from the fetal blood. Note that this membrane becomes very thin toward the end of pregnancy. Note also that at some sites nuclei in the syncytiotrophoblast form syncytial knots. These aggregations of nuclei break off and enter the maternal circulation. Some of them may lodge in the capillaries of the maternal lungs where they are rapidly destroyed by maternal enzymes. Fibrinoid material consists of fibrin and other substances. Formation of fibrinoid material mainly results from placental aging. (From Moore KL, Persaud TVN: The Developing Human, ed 5. Philadelphia, WB Saunders, 1993.)

the uterus during pregnancy decrease uteroplacental blood flow slightly, but they do not force significant amounts of blood out of the intervillous space. Consequently oxygen transfer to the fetus is decreased during uterine contractions, but the process does not stop.

Placental Membrane (Barrier)

This composite membrane *consists of the extrafetal tissues* separating the maternal and fetal blood (Figs. 4–6 and 4–7). Until about 20 weeks, it consists of four layers: (1) syncytiotrophoblast, (2) cytotrophoblast, (3) connective tissue in the villus, and (4) endothelium of the fetal capillaries.

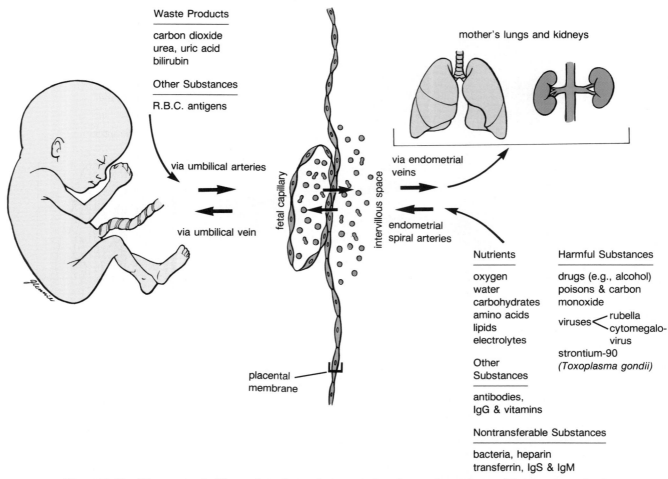

Figure 4-7. Diagrammatic illustration of transfer across the placental membrane (also inappropriately known as the placental barrier). The tissues across which transport of substances between the mother and fetus occurs collectively constitute the placental membrane. Note that this composite membrane is composed entirely of tissues of fetal origin: cytotrophoblast, syncytiotrophoblast, stroma (connective tissue) in the villus, and the endothelium of the fetus capillary (see also Figs. 4–5 and 4–6). Note that many harmful substances in the maternal blood in the intervillous space cross the placental membrane (e.g., alcohol and drugs) and enter the fetal circulation. Some of them cause congenital anomalies, e.g., fetal alcohol syndrome (see Fig. 5–11). Not all substances cross the placental membrane (e.g., bacteria). (Modified from Moore KL, Persaud TVN: The Developing Human, ed 5. Philadelphia, WB Saunders, 1993.)

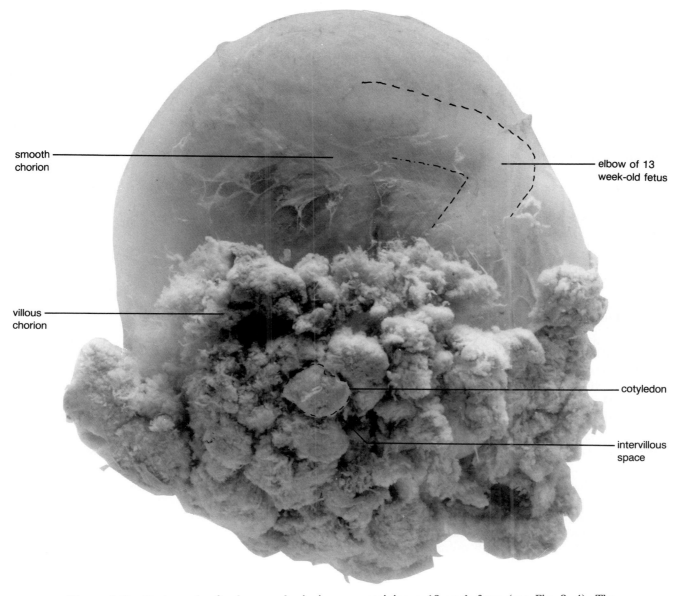

smooth
chorion

elbow of 13
week-old fetus

villous
chorion

cotyledon

intervillous
space

Figure 4-8. Photograph of a human chorionic sac containing a 13-week fetus (see Fig. 3-4). The smooth chorion (chorion laeve) forms when the chorionic villi degenerate and disappear from this area of the chorionic sac (see Fig. 4-1). The villous chorion (chorion frondosum) is where chorionic villi persist and form the fetal part of the placenta. In situ the cotyledons were attached to the decidua basalis and the intervillous space was filled with maternal blood (see Figs. 4-4 and 4-5).

Changes occur in the villi that result in the cytotrophoblast in the branch villi becoming attenuated. Eventually it disappears over large areas of the villi leaving only thin patches of syncytiotrophoblast (Fig. 4–6C). As a result, the placental membrane in near-term placentas consists of three layers only in most places.

Although the placental membrane is often called the *placental barrier,* this is an inappropriate term because there are only a few compounds, endogenous or exogenous, that are unable to pass through the placental membrane in detectable amounts. The placental membrane acts as a barrier only when the molecule has a certain size, configuration, and charge (e.g., heparin). Some metabolites, toxins, and hormones, though present in the maternal circulation, do not pass through the placental membrane in sufficient concentrations to affect the embryo/fetus. Most drugs and other substances present in the maternal plasma pass through the placental membrane and are found in the fetal plasma.

PARTURITION

Parturition (L. *parturitio,* childbirth) is the birth process during which the fetus, placenta, and fetal membranes are expelled from the mother's reproductive tract (Fig. 4–9). **Labor** is the sequence of involuntary *uterine contractions* that result in dilation of the cervix and delivery of the fetus and placenta from the uterus.

Stages of Labor

Labor (L. toil or suffering) is the process that is involved during the birth of a child that facilitates parturition. There are four stages, as follows (Fig. 4–9).

The first stage of labor (dilation stage) begins when there is objective evidence of progressive dilation of the cervix. This occurs when the onset of *regular contractions of the uterus occur* less than 10 minutes apart. The first stage ends with complete dilation of the cervix. This stage is by far the most time consuming of the labor process. The average duration is about 12 hours for first pregnancies (nulliparous patients, or *primigravidas*), and about 7 hours for women who have had a child previously (multiparous patients, or *multigravidas*). However, there are wide variations.

The second stage of labor (expulsion stage) begins when the cervix is fully dilated and ends with delivery of the baby. During this stage the *amniochorionic membrane* (fused amnion and smooth chorion) ruptures and *the fetus descends through the vagina* and is delivered (Fig. 4–9E). As soon as the fetus is outside the mother, it is called a newborn infant (or neonate). The average duration of this stage for primigravidas is 50 minutes, and 20 minutes for multigravidas. Uterine contractions begin again shortly after the baby is born.

The third stage of labor (placental stage) begins as soon as the baby is born and ends when the placenta and membranes are expelled (Fig. 4–9H). The duration of this stage is 15 minutes in about 90 per cent of pregnancies. *Retraction of the uterus reduces the area of placental attachment;* thus, the placenta and fetal membranes separate from the uterine wall and are expelled through the vagina. After delivery of the baby, the uterus continues to contract. A *hematoma* soon forms deep to the placenta and separates it from the uterine wall (Fig. 4–9G).

The fourth stage of labor (recovery stage) begins as soon as the placenta and fetal membranes are expelled. This stage lasts about two hours. The myometrial contractions constrict the spiral arteries that formerly supplied blood to the intervillous space (Fig. 4–4). This prevents excessive uterine bleeding.

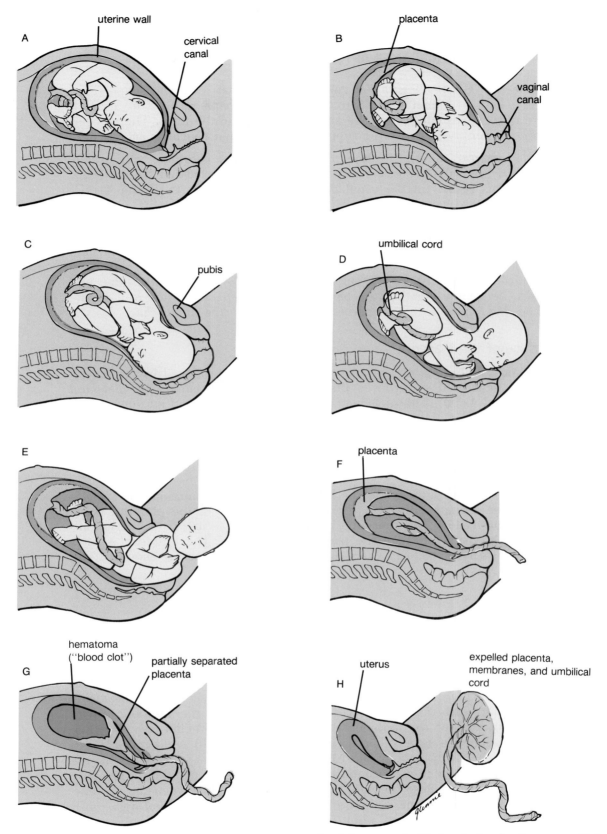

Figure 4–9. The process of birth or parturition. *A* and *B,* The cervix of the uterus is dilating during the first stage of labor. *C* to *E,* The amniochorionic membrane ruptures and the fetus passes through the cervix and vagina and is delivered during the second stage of labor. *F* and *G,* The uterus contracts during the third stage of labor and the placenta separates from the uterine wall. This results in bleeding and the formation of a large hematoma between the uterine wall and placenta. *H,* As soon as the placenta and membranes are expelled, the recovery or fourth stage of labor begins. The uterus contracts which constricts the endometrial arteries and prevents excessive bleeding.

PLACENTA AND FETAL MEMBRANES AFTER BIRTH

A full-term placenta (Gr. *plakuos,* a flat cake) commonly has a discoid shape (Figs. 4–10 to 4–12), with a diameter of 15 to 20 cm and a thickness of 2 to 3 cm. It weighs 500 to 600 gm, usually about one sixth the weight of the fetus. The margins of the placenta are continuous with the ruptured amniotic and chorionic sacs.

VARIATIONS IN PLACENTAL SHAPE. As the placenta develops, chorionic villi usually persist only where the villous chorion is in contact with the decidua basalis (Figs. 4–1 and 4–8). This results in the usual discoid placenta (Figs. 4–10 and 4–11). When villi persist elsewhere, several variations in placental shape occur: *accessory placenta* (Fig. 4–15), bidiscoid placenta, diffuse placenta, and horseshoe placenta. Although there are variations in the size and shape of the placenta, most of them are of little physiologic or clinical significance. However, examination of the placenta may provide information about the causes of (1) placental dysfunction, (2) intrauterine growth retardation (IUGR), (3) neonatal illness, and (4) infant death. Placental studies can also determine whether the placenta is complete. Retention of a cotyledon or an accessory placenta in the uterus may lead to *uterine hemorrhage.*

Maternal Surface of the Placenta

The characteristic cobblestone appearance of this surface is produced by the *cotyledons,* which are separated by grooves that were formerly occupied by *placental septa* (Figs. 4–5 and 4–10). The surface of the cotyledons is covered by thin grayish shreds of decidua basalis that separated with the placenta. Most of the decidua is temporarily retained in the uterus and is shed with subsequent uterine bleeding.

Fetal Surface of the Placenta

The umbilical cord usually attaches to the fetal surface and its amniotic covering is continuous with the amnion adherent to the chorionic plate of the placenta (Figs. 4–2, 4–4, 4–5, and 4–11). The chorionic vessels radiating to and from the umbilical cord are clearly visible through the transparent amnion. The *umbilical vessels* branch on the fetal surface to form *chorionic vessels,* which enter the chorionic villi (Figs. 4–4 to 4–6).

UMBILICAL CORD

The attachment of the umbilical cord, which connects the embryo/fetus to the placenta, is usually near the center of the fetal surface of this organ (Fig. 4–11), but it may be found at any point. For example, insertion of it near the placental margin produces a *battledore placenta* (Fig. 4–12) and its attachment to the membranes is called a *velamentous insertion of the cord* (Fig. 4–13). As the amniotic cavity enlarges the amnion enfolds the umbilical cord, forming its epithelial covering (Fig. 4–2). The umbilical cord is usually 1 to 2 cm in diameter and 30 to 90 cm in length (average 55 cm). Excessively long or short cords are uncommon. Long cords have a tendency to prolapse and/or to coil around the fetus. Prompt recognition of *prolapse of the cord* is important because the cord may be compressed between the presenting body part of the fetus and the mother's bony pelvis. This causes *fetal hypoxia.* If anoxia persists for more than five minutes, the baby's brain may be damaged, producing mental retardation.

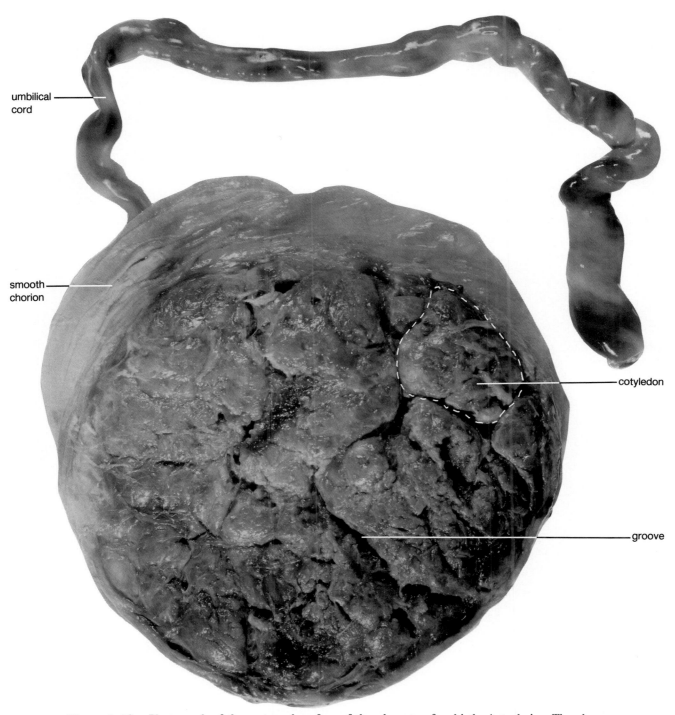

umbilical cord

smooth chorion

cotyledon

groove

Figure 4-10. Photograph of the maternal surface of the placenta after birth. Actual size. The characteristic cobblestone appearance of this surface is caused by 15 to 20 cotyledons. Each cotyledon is composed of two or more stem villi and their many branches (see Figs. 4-4 and 4-5). The cotyledons are separated by grooves which in situ were occupied by placental septa. The external surfaces of the cotyledons are covered with remnants of the decidua basalis which separated from the uterus during parturition. The whitish appearance of some of the cotyledons is due to excessive fibrinoid formation (Fig. 4-6C) that causes infarction of portions of the villi.

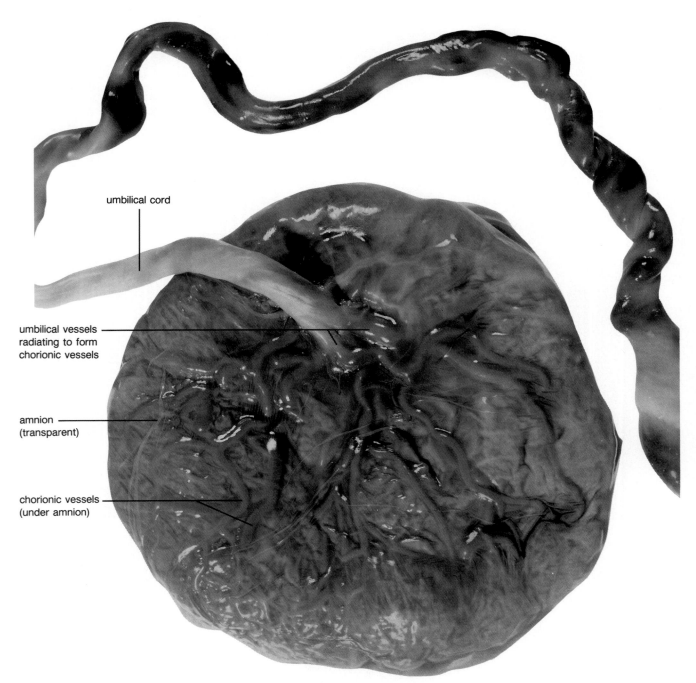

umbilical cord

umbilical vessels
radiating to form
chorionic vessels

amnion
(transparent)

chorionic vessels
(under amnion)

Figure 4–11. Photograph of the fetal surface of the placenta after birth. The umbilical cord is attached to this surface. The attachment is usually eccentric as in this specimen. A number of large arteries and veins, the chorionic vessels, may be seen converging toward the umbilical cord, where they form the umbilical vessels. The chorionic vessels are covered by amnion that is continuous with the epithelial covering of the umbilical cord (see Figs. 4–2 and 4–6).

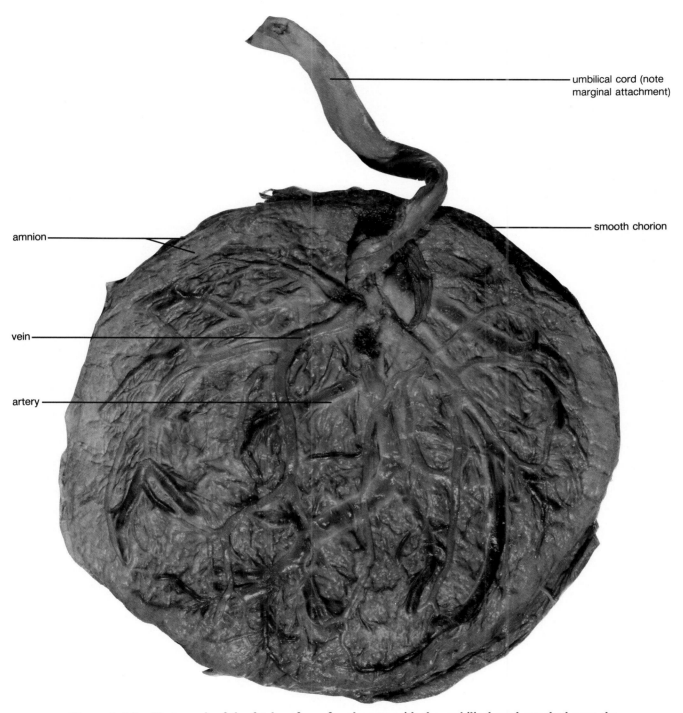

umbilical cord (note
marginal attachment)

smooth chorion

amnion

vein

artery

Figure 4–12. Photograph of the fetal surface of a placenta with the umbilical cord attached near the margin of the placenta. Usually the cord attaches near the center of the placenta (Fig. 4–11). A placenta with a marginal attachment of the cord is sometimes called a battledore placenta because of its resemblance to the bat used in the medieval game of battledore and shuttlecock.

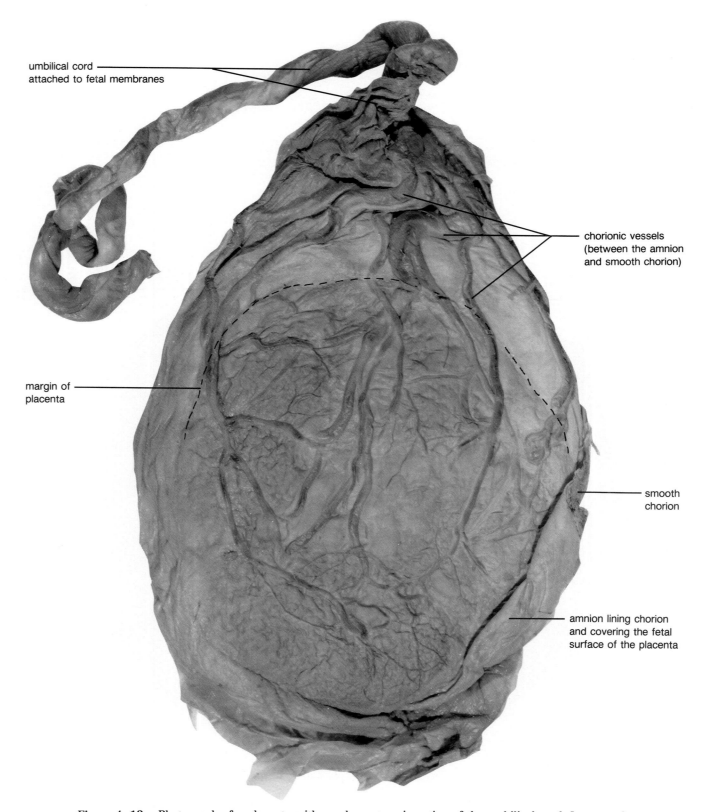

umbilical cord
attached to fetal membranes

chorionic vessels
(between the amnion
and smooth chorion)

margin of
placenta

smooth
chorion

amnion lining chorion
and covering the fetal
surface of the placenta

Figure 4–13. Photograph of a placenta with a velamentous insertion of the umbilical cord. In unusual cases, as here, the cord does not attach to the placenta but inserts onto the smooth chorion away from the placenta and chorionic villi. The umbilical vessels leave the umbilical cord and run between the amnion and chorion to reach the placenta and chorionic villi. The blood vessels are easily torn in this location, which results in the loss of fetal blood.

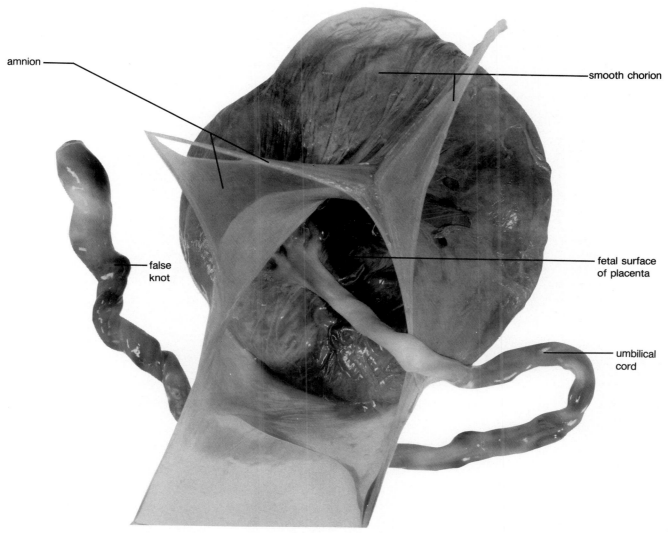

amnion

smooth chorion

false knot

fetal surface of placenta

umbilical cord

Figure 4-14. Photograph of the fetal membranes and the fetal surface of the placenta. The amnion and smooth chorion are arranged to show that they are fused and continuous with the margin of the placenta (see also Figs. 4-4 and 4-5). Observe the false knots in the umbilical cord that develop when the umbilical vessels form loops. False knots are of no clinical significance. A true knot in the cord can cause the death of the fetus if it tightens and obstructs blood flow (Fig. 4-16A).

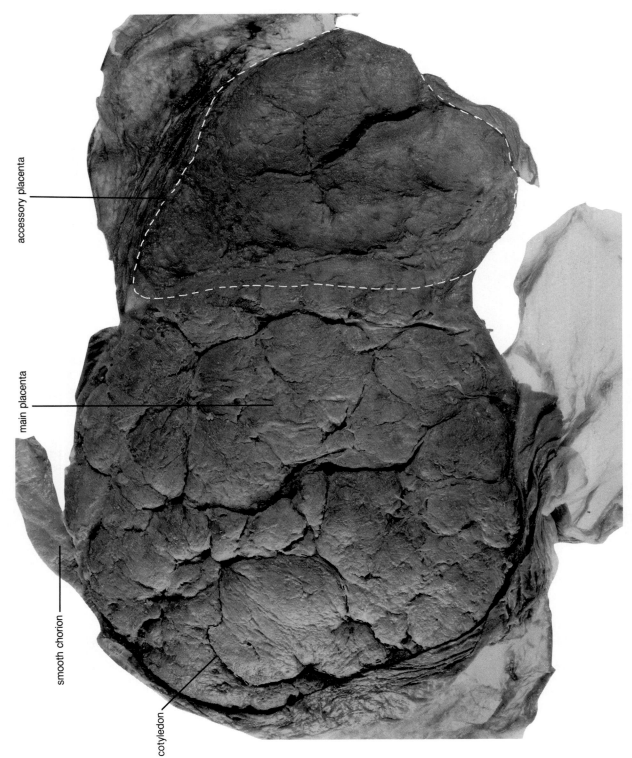

accessory placenta

main placenta

smooth chorion

cotyledon

Figure 4–15. Photograph of the maternal surface of an odd-shaped placenta due to the presence of an accessory placenta. The additional placenta developed from chorionic villi that persisted close to the normal placenta. It resembles the fused placentas of twins except that only one umbilical cord is attached to it.

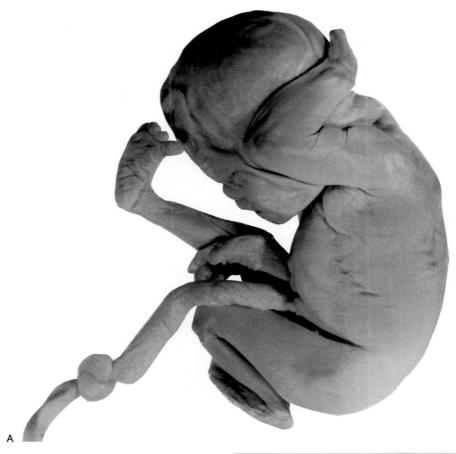

Figure 4–16. *A*, Photograph of a 20-week fetus with a true knot in its umbilical cord. Note that the diameter of the cord is greater near the fetus, indicating that blood was unable to enter or leave the fetus. Undoubtedly, the fetus died and aborted spontaneously due to a lack of oxygen (anoxia). *B*, Photograph of a fetus with the amniotic band syndrome. This stillborn has multiple anomalies including encephalocele, facial clefting, and a lateral abdominal wall defect with exterioration of the thoracic and abdominal contents due to thoracoabdominal schisis (failure of embryonic fusion of the abdominal wall). The right upper limb is rudimentary. Note the short umbilical cord with attachment of the placenta to the intestine. The primary event is believed to be a vascular disruption with secondary adhesion and disruption of the amnion. (Courtesy of Dr. A.E. Chudley, Children's Centre, Winnipeg, Canada.)

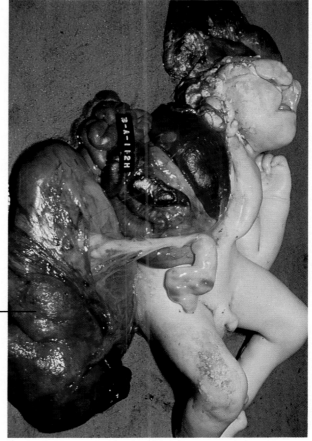

placenta

B

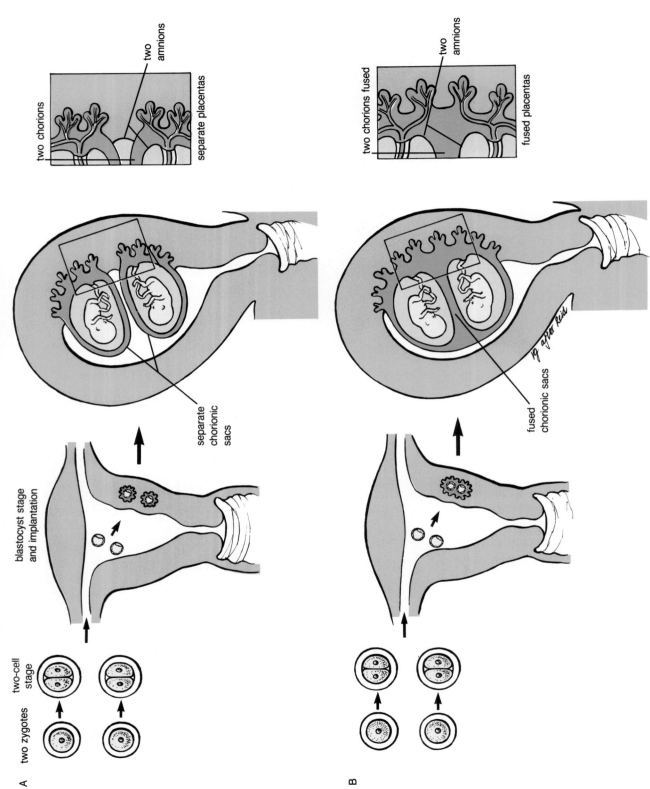

Figure 4-17. Drawings showing how the most common type of twins, dizygotic (or fraternal) twins, develop. They result from the fertilization of two ova by different sperms which form two zygotes. They always have two amnions and two chorionic sacs and their placentas may be separate or fused. The twins may be of the same sex or different sexes and are no more alike than brothers or sisters born at different times.

A, The two blastocysts have implanted separately in the endometrium. *B,* The blastocysts have implanted close together and their placentas have fused. Similarly the walls of their chorionic sacs have fused. In some cases the blood vessels of the two placentas anastomose (as shown in Fig. 4–18) which results in erythrocyte mosaicism, i.e., the twins possess red blood cells of two different types.

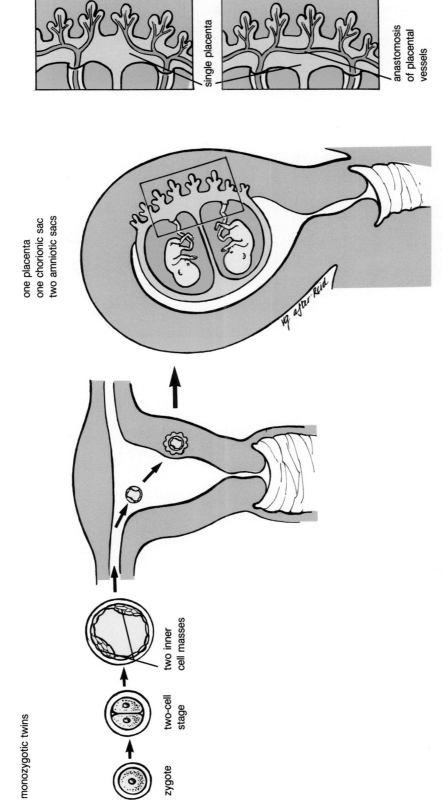

single placenta

anastomosis of placental vessels

monozygotic twins

zygote

two-cell stage

two inner cell masses

one placenta
one chorionic sac
two amniotic sacs

fig. after Reid

Figure 4-18. Drawings showing how monozygotic (or identical) twins develop from one zygote. They result from the division of blastomeres at various stages of cleavage (see Figs. 1–1 to 1–3). The separation may occur at the two-cell to morula stage, in which case two blastocysts develop and implant separately. Each embryo has its own placenta and chorionic sac, similar to that which occurs in dizygotic twinning (Fig. 4–17). In these cases, it is not possible to determine from the membranes alone whether the twins are monozygotic (MZ) or dizygotic (DZ). In most cases, MZ twinning occurs at the early blastocyst stage. The inner cell mass, as shown, splits into two separate groups of embryonic cells. The two embryos that develop have separate amnions but a common chorionic sac and placenta (see also Fig. 4–19B). Often, there is anastomosis of the placental vessels, but this is of no consequence because they have the same blood groups.

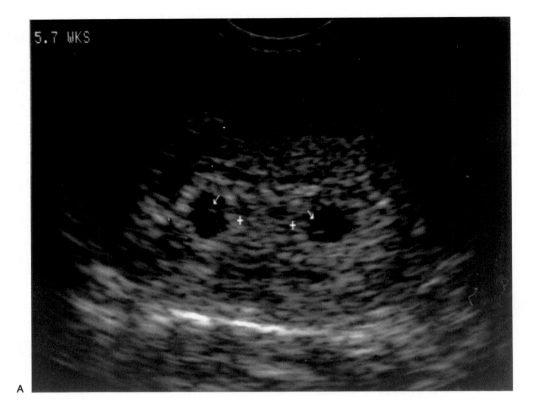

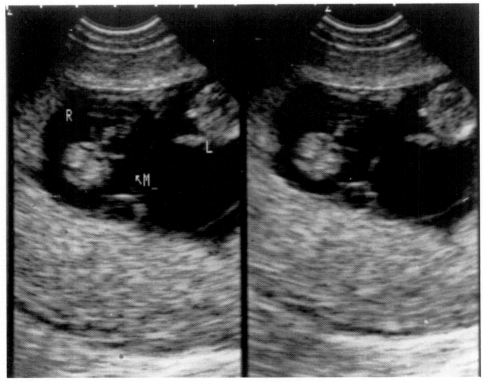

Figure 4–19. Ultrasound scans of pregnant uteri. *A,* Diamniotic/dichorionic twin gestation at 5.7 weeks. (3.7 weeks after fertilization). The *arrows* indicate the yolk sacs of the dizygotic twins in their chorionic sacs. *B,* Diamniotic/monochorionic twin gestation at 11 weeks (9 weeks after fertilization). The fused amnions (M) separate the monozygotic fetuses (R and L). (Courtesy of Dr. Lyndon M. Hill, Department of Obstetrics and Gynecology, Division of Maternal-Fetal Medicine, University of Pittsburgh, Pittsburgh, PA.)

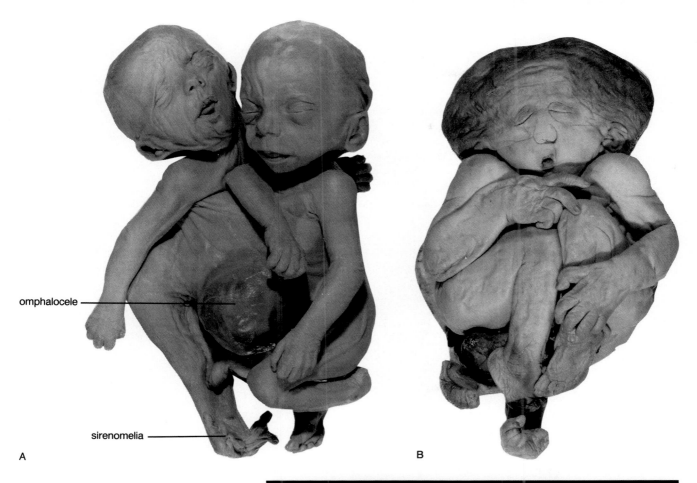

omphalocele

sirenomelia

A

B

Figure 4-20. Conjoined ("Siamese") twins. *A*, Fusion in the thoracoabdominal regions. A large omphalocoele containing common intestines and covered with amnion is present. The lower limbs of one twin are fused, a condition known as sirenomelia. Both twins have large malformed ears. *B*, Complete fusion. Multiple congenital anomalies are present. *C*, In this uncommon case, separation of the embryonic disc occurred early in the third week as the primitive streak was developing. The twins share a placenta and have common chorionic and amniotic sacs. It has been estimated that about once in every 40 monozygotic twin pregnancies, the twinning is incomplete and conjoined twins develop. If the fusion is extensive, as in these cases, it is impossible to separate the infants. (Part *C* courtesy of Dr. Susan Phillips, Department of Pathology, Health Science Centre, Winnipeg, Manitoba, Canada.)

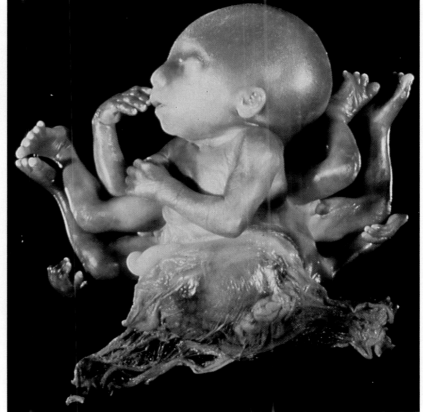

C

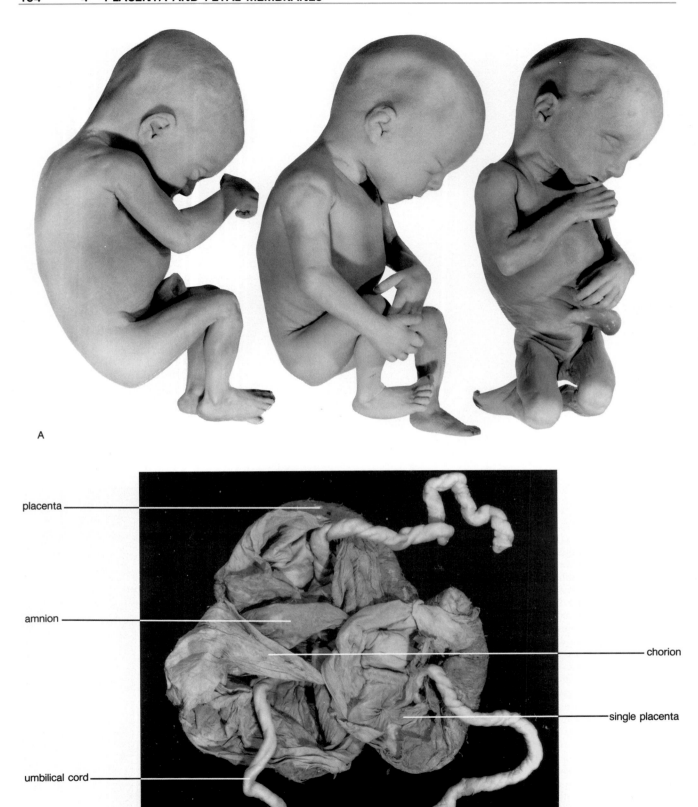

Figure 4–21. Photographs of triplets with their placentas and fetal membranes. Triplets may develop from one, two, or three zygotes. Examination of the placentas and membranes reveals that the two fetuses on the left were identical and the one on the right was a singleton. The diamniotic/monochorionic placenta is on the left and the single placenta is on the right. Thus, these three fetuses developed from two zygotes. In recent years multiple births have occurred more frequently in mothers given fertility drugs for ovulatory failure.

5

CONGENITAL ANOMALIES OR BIRTH DEFECTS

Birth defects or congenital anomalies may be structural, functional, metabolic, behavioral, or hereditary. More than 20 per cent of infant deaths in North America are attributed to birth defects. Major structural anomalies (e.g., cleft lip and spina bifida cystica) are observed in about 3 per cent of newborn infants. Additional anomalies can be detected after birth; thus the incidence reaches about 6 per cent in 2-year-olds and 8 per cent in 5-year-olds.

Anomalies may be single or multiple and of major or minor clinical significance. Single *minor anomalies* are present in about 14 per cent of newborns. These defects (e.g., of the external ear) are of no serious medical or cosmetic significance, but they indicate to the clinician the possible presence of associated clinically significant anomalies.

Ninety per cent of infants with three or more minor anomalies also have one or more major defects. Of the 3 per cent born with clinically significant congenital anomalies, 0.7 per cent have multiple major anomalies. Most of these infants die during infancy (e.g., those with trisomy 18 [Fig. 5–7]). Major developmental defects are much more common in early embryos (10 to 15 per cent), but most of them abort spontaneously. Chromosome abnormalities are present in 50 to 60 per cent of spontaneously aborted early embryos.

The causes of congenital anomalies are often divided into *genetic factors* (e.g., chromosome abnormalities) and *environmental factors,* such as drugs and viruses (Figs. 5–1 and 5–2). However, many common congenital anomalies are caused by genetic and environmental factors acting together. This is called *multifactorial inheritance.* For 50 to 60 per cent of congenital anomalies, the causes are unknown (Fig. 5–1).

ANOMALIES CAUSED BY GENETIC FACTORS

Numerically, *genetic factors are the most important causes of congenital anomalies* (Fig. 5–1; Tables 5–1 and 5–2). It has been estimated that they cause about a third of all birth defects and nearly 85 per cent of all those with known causes. Any mechanism as complex as mitosis or meiosis[1] may occasionally malfunction. Thus, *chromosomal aberrations are common* and are present in 6 to 7 per cent of zygotes. Many of these primordial cells never undergo normal cleavage (mitosis) and become blastocysts. *In vitro studies of early embryos* (cleaving human zygotes) less than 5

---

[1] The special type of cell division occurring in the germ cells by which gametes (ova or sperms) containing the haploid chromosome number (23) are produced from diploid cells containing 46 chromosomes.

days old have revealed a high incidence of abnormalities. Many defective zygotes, blastocysts, and early embryos abort spontaneously during the first three weeks and the overall frequency of chromosome abnormalities in them is at least 50 per cent.

Two kinds of change occur in chromosome complements: numerical and structural, and they may affect the sex chromosomes and/or the autosomes.[2] In some cases, both kinds of chromosome are affected. People with *numerical chromosome abnormalities* usually have characteristic phenotypes (e.g., the physical characteristics of Down syndrome [Fig. 5–3; Tables 5–1 and 5–2]), and they often look more like other people with the same chromosome abnormality than like their own siblings (brothers or sisters). This characteristic appearance results from genetic imbalance.

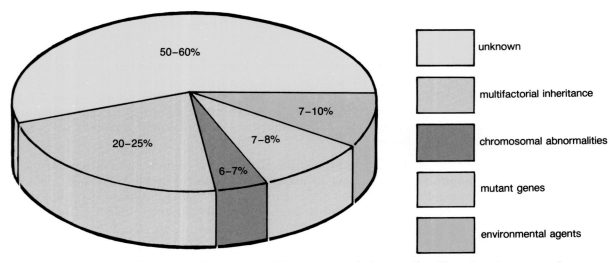

Figure 5–1. Graphic illustration of the causes of human congenital anomalies. Note that the causes of most anomalies are unknown and that 25 per cent of them are caused by a combination of genetic and environmental factors (multifactorial inheritance).

TABLE 5–1. TRISOMY OF THE AUTOSOMES

Chromosomal Aberration/Syndrome	Incidence	Usual Characteristics
Trisomy 21 or Down syndrome*	1 : 800	Mental deficiency; brachycephaly, flat nasal bridge; upward slant to palpebral fissures; protruding tongue; simian crease, clinodactyly of 5th digit; congenital heart defects.
Trisomy 18 syndrome†	1 : 8000	Mental deficiency; growth retardation; prominent occiput; short sternum; ventricular septal defect; micrognathia; low-set malformed ears; flexed digits, hypoplastic nails; rocker-bottom feet.
Trisomy 13 syndrome†	1 : 25000	Mental deficiency; severe central nervous system malformations; sloping forehead; malformed ears, scalp defects; microphthalmia; bilateral cleft lip and/or palate; polydactyly; posterior prominence of the heels.

* The importance of this disorder in the overall problem of mental retardation is indicated by the fact that persons with Down syndrome represent ten to 15 per cent of institutionalized mental defectives. *The incidence of trisomy 21 at fertilization is greater than at birth,* but 75 per cent of the embryos are spontaneously aborted and at least 20 per cent are stillborn.
† Infants with this syndrome rarely survive beyond six months.
(Adapted from Moore KL and Persaud TVN: *The Developing Human,* ed 5. Philadelphia, WB Saunders, 1993.)

---

[2] Autosomes are chromosomes other than sex chromosomes. There are 22 pairs of autosomes in the human karyotype (chromosome constitution).

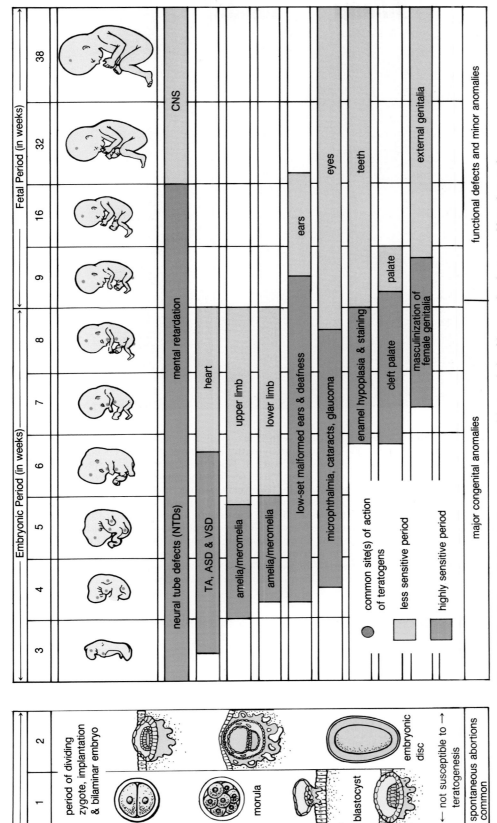

Figure 5–2. Schematic illustration showing the critical periods of human development. Note that each part or organ of the embryo has a critical period when development may be disrupted, resulting in major congenital anomalies. Thereafter is a period when environmental agents (e.g., drugs and viruses) may cause minor anomalies and functional disturbances (e.g., mental retardation). TA, Truncus arteriosus; ASD, atrial septal defect; VSD, ventricular septal defect; NTDs, neural tube defects, e.g., spina bifida (see Figs. 13–14 to 13–18).

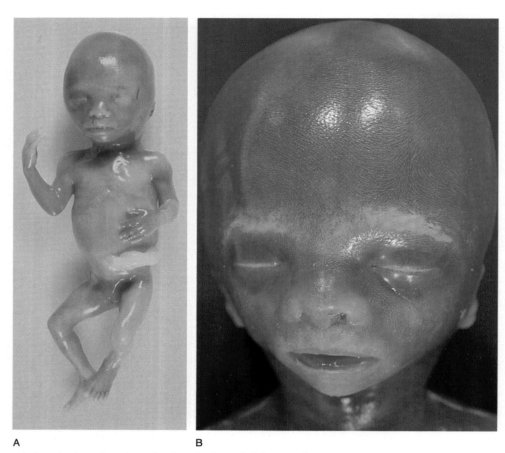

A   B

Figure 5–3. *A,* Anterior view of a female fetus (16.5 weeks) with Down syndrome. See Table 5–1 for a list of the usual characteristics associated with this type of trisomy of the autosomes. *B,* Anterior view of the craniofacial region of a fetus with Down syndrome (16 weeks). Note the minimal dysmorphic features. *C,* Lateral view of the craniofacial region of the fetus. Note the brachycephaly (shortness of the head) and small ears. *D,* Hand of the fetus. Note the single, transverse palmar, flexion ("simian") crease and the clinodactyly (incurving) of the fifth digit. Not all persons with Down syndrome have transverse palmar creases. About three quarters of fetuses with Down syndrome (trisomy 21) are lost by spontaneous abortion, usually in the first trimester. The frequency of Down syndrome increases with maternal age (Table 5–2). In most cases the chromosome aberration results from nondisjunction of the number 21 chromosomes during oogenesis rather than spermatogenesis. (Part *A* courtesy of Dr. D.K. Kalousek, Professor, Department of Pathology, University of British Columbia, Vancouver, B.C., Canada. Part *D* courtesy of Dr. A.E. Chudley, Professor of Pediatrics and Child Health, Children's Centre, Winnipeg, Manitoba, Canada.)

TABLE 5–2.   INCIDENCE OF DOWN SYNDROME IN NEWBORN INFANTS*

Maternal Age* (Years)	Incidence
20–24	1:1400
25–29	1:1100
30–34	1:700
35	1:350
37	1:225
39	1:140
41	1:85
43	1:50
45+	1:25

* Based on data from several sources. Figures have been rounded and are approximate.
(Adapted from Moore KL and Persaud TVN: *The Developing Human,* ed 5. Philadelphia, WB Saunders, 1993.)

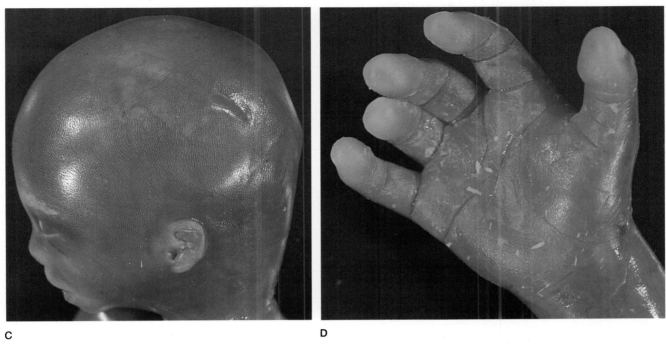

C

D

Figure 5-3. *Continued.*

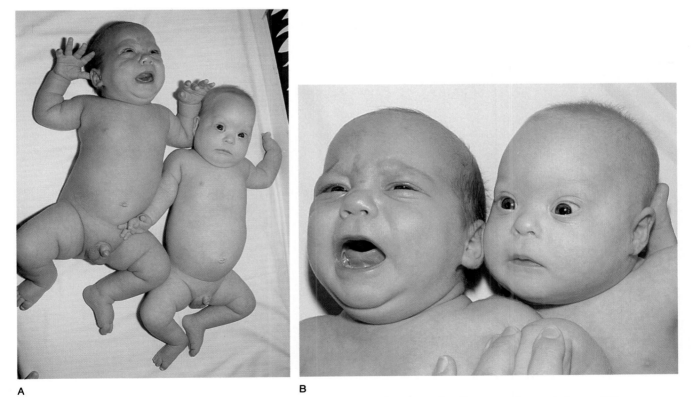

A

B

Figure 5-4. Dizygotic (fraternal) male twins that are discordant for Down syndrome (trisomy 21). *A,* Anterior view of the twins. The one on the right is smaller and hypotonic compared with the unaffected twin. The twin on the right developed from a zygote that contained an extra 21 chromosome. *B,* Close-up of their faces. Note the characteristic facial features of Down syndrome in the infant on the right (upslanting palpebral fissures, epicanthal folds and flat nasal bridge). (Courtesy of Dr. A.E. Chudley, Professor of Pediatrics and Child Health, Children's Centre, Winnipeg, Manitoba, Canada).

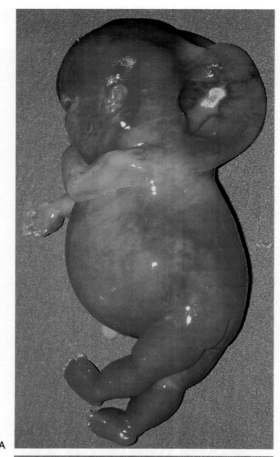

A

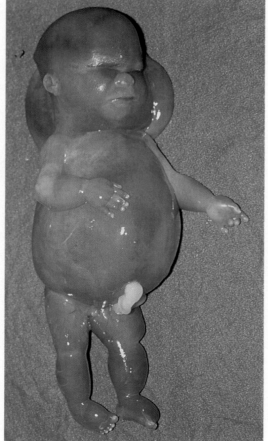

B

Figure 5-5. *A,* Female fetus (16 weeks) with Turner syndrome and a chromosome constitution of 45,X (sometimes written as 45,XO). She had no second sex chromosome, either X or Y. Note the excessive accumulation of watery fluid (hydrops) and the large cystic hygroma (cystic lymphangioma) in the cervical region. The hygroma causes the loose neck skin and webbing seen postnatally (Fig. 5-6B). *A,* Lateral view. *B,* Anterolateral view. This chromosomal abnormality is present in 1.5 per cent of all conceptuses and accounts for about 18 per cent of all chromosomally abnormal spontaneous abortions. (Courtesy of Dr. A.E. Chudley, Professor of Pediatrics and Child Health, Children's Centre, Winnipeg, Manitoba, Canada).

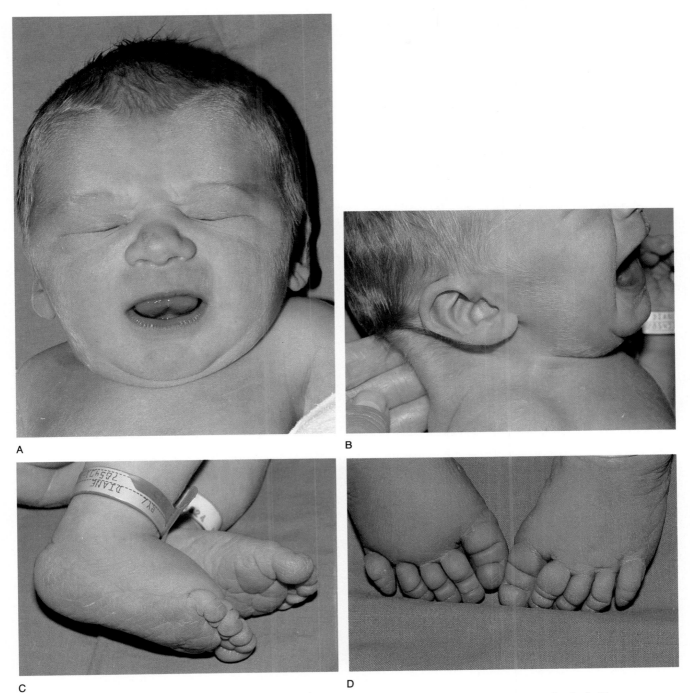

Figure 5–6. *A,* Face of a female infant with Turner syndrome (45,X chromosome constitution). Note the short neck. *B,* Lateral view of the infant's head and neck, showing the short neck, low set ears, and redundant skin at the back of the neck. These infants have gonadal dysgenesis (usually streak gonads). *C,* Photograph of the infant's feet showing the characteristic lymphedema, a useful diagnostic sign. *D,* Lymphedema of the toes, a condition that usually leads to nail hypoplasia. In older females with this chromosome abnormality, there is absence of sexual maturation. (Courtesy of Dr. A.E. Chudley, Professor of Pediatrics and Child Health, Children's Centre, Winnipeg, Manitoba, Canada).

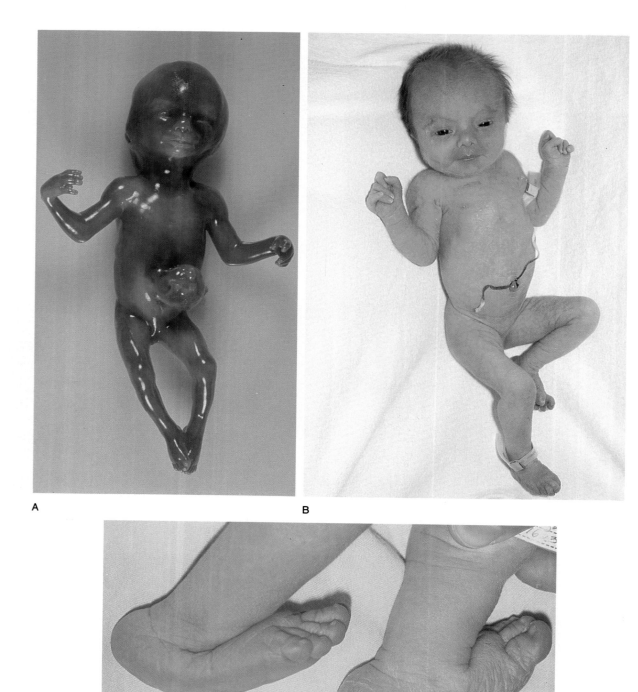

A

B

C

Figure 5–7. Trisomy 18 has an incidence of about 1 in 8000 births. The incidence at fertilization is higher, but about 95 per cent of trisomy 18 fetuses are spontaneously aborted. The features of trisomy 18 always include mental retardation and failure to thrive, and often include a heart anomaly (Table 5–1). Postnatal survival for more than a few months is uncommon. Most affected fetuses and neonates are female. Late maternal age is a causative factor. *A,* Female fetus (15.5 weeks) with trisomy 18. Note the low-set malformed ears and the abnormal position of the hands. *B,* Female neonate with trisomy 18. Note the growth retardation, clenched fists with characteristic positioning of the fingers (second and fifth digits overlapping the third and fourth), short sternum, and narrow pelvis. *C,* The feet of another trisomy 18 infant showing the characteristic rocker-bottom appearance due to the vertical position of the tali (ankle bones). Also observe the prominent calcanei (heel bones). (Part *A* courtesy of Dr. D.K. Kalousek, Professor, Department of Pathology, University of British Columbia, Vancouver, B.C., Canada. Part *C* courtesy of Dr. A.E. Chudley, Professor of Pediatrics and Child Health, Children's Centre, Winnipeg, Manitoba, Canada).

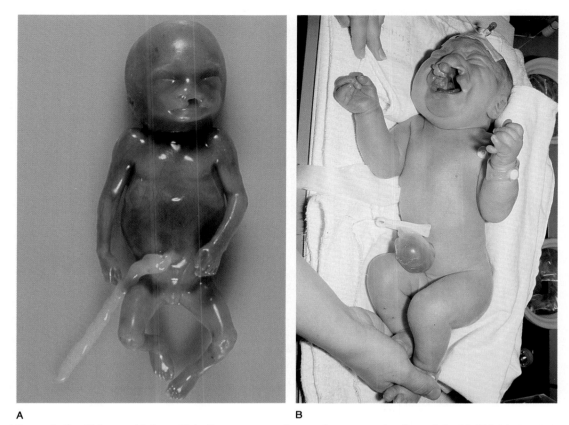

A   B

Figure 5-8. Trisomy 13 is a clinically severe syndrome that occurs in about 1 in 25,000 births. It is lethal in almost all cases by the age of 6 months. Associated with late maternal age, the extra 13 chromosome arises from nondisjunction during the first division of maternal meiosis. *A*, Male fetus (15.5 weeks). Observe the severe cleft lip and low-set ears. *B*, Female neonate with trisomy 13. Note particularly the bilateral cleft lip, low-set malformed ear, and polydactyly (extra digits). A small omphalocele (herniation of viscera into the umbilical cord) is also present. For other defects characteristic of this syndrome, see Table 5-1. (Part *A* courtesy of Dr. D.K. Kalousek, Professor, Department of Pathology, University of British Columbia, Vancouver, B.C., Canada. Part *B* courtesy of Dr. A.E. Chudley, Professor of Pediatrics and Child Health, Children's Centre, Winnipeg, Manitoba, Canada.)

Structural chromosome abnormalities result from **chromosome breakage** that is induced by various environmental factors, e.g., radiation, drugs, chemicals, and viruses. The type of abnormality that results depends upon what happens to the broken pieces of the chromosomes (Fig. 5-9). The only aberrations that are likely to be transmitted from parent to child are structural rearrangements, such as inversion and translocation (Thompson et al., 1991).

DELETION (Fig. 5-9*A*).   When a chromosome breaks, a portion of the chromosome may be lost. A partial terminal deletion from the short arm of chromosome number 5 causes the **cri du chat syndrome.** Affected infants have a weak, catlike cry, microcephaly, severe mental retardation, and congenital heart disease. A *ring chromosome* (Fig. 5-9*C*) is a type of deletion chromosome from which both ends have been lost, and the broken ends have rejoined to form a ring-shaped chromosome. These abnormal chromosomes have been described in persons with Turner syndrome, trisomy 18, and other abnormalities.

TRANSLOCATION (Fig. 5-9*E*).   This is the transfer of a piece of one chromosome to a nonhomologous chromosome. Translocation does not necessarily lead to abnormal development.

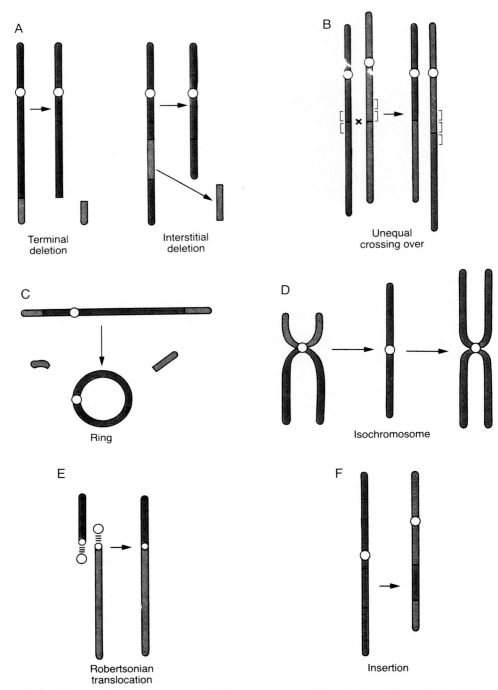

Figure 5–9. Structural rearrangements of chromosomes. *A,* Terminal and interstitial deletions, each generating an acentric fragment. *B,* Unequal crossing over between segments of homologous chromosomes or between sister chromatids (the duplicated or deleted segment is indicated by brackets). *C,* Ring chromosome with two acentric fragments. *D,* Generation of an isochromosome for the long arm of a chromosome. *E,* Robertsonian translocation between two acrocentric chromosomes. *F,* Insertion of a segment of one chromosome into a nonhomologous chromosome. (From Thompson MW, McInnes RR, and Willard HF: *Thompson and Thompson: Genetics in Medicine,* ed 5. Philadelphia, WB Saunders, 1991.)

DUPLICATION (Fig. 5–9B). This abnormality may be represented as a duplicated portion of a chromosome: (1) within a chromosome, (2) attached to a chromosome, or (3) as a separate fragment. *Duplications are more common than deletions and they are less harmful* because there is no loss of genetic material. Duplication may involve part of a gene, a whole gene, or a series of genes.

INVERSION. This is a chromosomal aberration in which a segment of a chromosome is reversed.

ISOCHROMOSOME (Fig. 5–9D). The abnormality results when the centromere divides transversely instead of longitudinally. It appears to be the *most common structural abnormality of the X chromosome*. Patients with this chromosomal abnormality are often short in stature and have other stigmata of the Turner syndrome.

Anomalies Caused by Mutant Genes

Probably 8 per cent of congenital anomalies are caused by mutant genes (Fig. 5–1). A *mutation* usually involves a loss or a change in the function of a gene. Because a random change is unlikely to lead to an improvement in development, most mutations are deleterious and some are lethal. The mutation rate can be increased by a number of environmental agents, e.g., large doses of radiation and some chemicals, especially carcinogenic (cancer-inducing) ones.

Examples of *dominantly inherited congenital anomalies* are **achondroplasia** and some types of polydactyly. Other anomalies are attributed to *autosomal recessive inheritance*, e.g., congenital adrenal hyperplasia (see Fig. 10–18) and microcephaly.

Thanatophoric dysplasia or dwarfism (Fig. 5–10) is probably the most frequent lethal congenital skeletal dysplasia. As the limbs are extremely short, this condition is sometimes misdiagnosed as achondroplasia. The thorax is very narrow in all dimensions and in neonates respiratory distress contributes to early death.

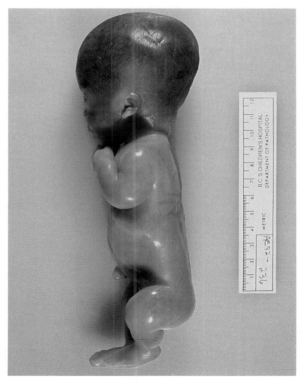

Figure 5–10. Male fetus (18 weeks) with thanatophoric dwarfism or dysplasia, showing shortening of the limbs, a large head, and depressed nasal bridge. The most likely cause of this condition is a dominant mutation. (Courtesy of Dr. D.K. Kalousek, Professor, Department of Pathology, University of British Columbia, Vancouver, B.C., Canada).

ANOMALIES CAUSED BY ENVIRONMENTAL FACTORS

Although the human embryo is well protected in the uterus, certain environmental agents called **teratogens** may cause developmental disruptions following maternal exposure to them (Table 5–3). A teratogen is any agent that can produce a congenital anomaly or raise the incidence of an anomaly in the population. Environmental factors, such as infection and drugs, may simulate genetic conditions; e.g., when two or more children of normal parents are affected (Holmes, 1992).

Environmental factors cause 7 to 10 per cent of congenital anomalies (Fig. 5–1). Because biochemical differentiation precedes morphologic differentiation, the period during which structures are sensitive to interference often precedes the stage of their visible development by a few days. Teratogens do not appear to be effective in causing anomalies until cellular differentiation has begun. However, their early actions may cause death of the embryo.

CRITICAL PERIODS IN HUMAN DEVELOPMENT (Fig. 5–2). The organs and parts of an embryo are most sensitive to teratogenic agents during periods of rapid differentiation. The stage of development of an embryo when a teratogenic agent is present determines its susceptibility to a teratogen. The most critical period in development is when cell division, cell differentiation, and morphogenesis are at their peak.

Human Teratogens and Congenital Anomalies

Awareness that certain agents can disrupt embryonic development offers the opportunity to prevent some congenital anomalies (Table 5–3). For example, if women are made aware of the harmful effects of drugs (e.g., alcohol), environmental chemicals (e.g., PCBs) and viruses (e.g., rubella), most of them will not expose their embryos to these teratogenic agents.

Drugs as Teratogens

Drugs vary considerably in their teratogenicity. Some cause severe disruptions of development if administered during the organogenetic period (e.g., thalidomide causes severe limb defects and other anomalies). Other drugs produce mental and growth retardation and other anomalies if used excessively throughout development (e.g., alcohol [Fig. 5–11]).

The use of prescription and nonprescription drugs during pregnancy is surprisingly high. From 40 to 90 per cent of pregnant women consume at least one drug. Several studies have indicated that some pregnant women take an average of four drugs, excluding nutritional supplements, and about half of these women take them during the first trimester of pregnancy. Drug consumption also tends to be higher during the critical period of development among heavy smokers and heavy drinkers (Persaud, 1990).

Infectious Agents as Teratogens

Throughout prenatal life, the embryo and fetus are endangered by a variety of **microorganisms.** In most cases, the assault is resisted; in some cases, a spontaneous abortion or stillbirth occurs; in others, the infants are born with growth retardation, congenital anomalies, or neonatal diseases (Table 5–3). The microorganisms, especially *viruses,* cross the placental membrane and enter the fetal blood stream (see Fig. 4–7). The fetal blood-brain barrier also appears to offer little resistance to microorganisms, because there is a propensity for the central nervous system to be affected. The rubella virus is the prime example of an *infective teratogen.* The risk is about 20 per cent when maternal infection occurs during the first trimester. The usual features of *congenital rubella syndrome* are cataract (Fig. 5–12A), cardiac defects, and deafness. For other teratogenic effects of this and other viruses, see Table 5–3.

TABLE 5-3. TERATOGENS KNOWN TO CAUSE HUMAN BIRTH DEFECTS*

Agents	Most Common Congenital Anomalies
DRUGS	
Alcohol	*Fetal alcohol syndrome (FAS):* intrauterine growth retardation *(IUGR);* mental retardation, microcephaly; ocular anomalies; joint abnormalities; short palpebral fissures (Fig. 5–11).
Androgens and high doses of progestogens	Varying degrees of masculinization of female fetuses: ambiguous external genitalia resulting in labial fusion and clitoral hypertrophy (see Fig. 10–18).
Aminopterin	IUGR; skeletal defects; malformations of the central nervous system, notably meroanencephaly (most of the brain is absent).
Busulfan	Stunted growth; skeletal abnormalities; corneal opacities; cleft palate; hypoplasia of various organs.
Cocaine	IUGR; microcephaly; cerebral infarction; urogenital anomalies; neurobehavioral disturbances.
Diethylstilbesterol	Abnormalities of the uterus and vagina; cervical erosion and ridges.
Isotretinoin (13-cis-retinoic acid)	Craniofacial abnormalities; neural tube defects *(NTDs),* such as spina bifida cystica; cardiovascular defects.
Lithium carbonate	Various anomalies usually involving the heart and great vessels.
Methotrexate	Multiple malformations, especially skeletal, involving the face, skull, limbs, and vertebral column.
Phenytoin (Dilantin)	*Fetal hydantoin syndrome (FHS):* IUGR; microcephaly; mental retardation; ridged metopic suture; inner epicanthal folds; eyelid ptosis; broad depressed nasal bridge; phalangeal hypoplasia.
Tetracycline	Stained teeth; hypoplasia of enamel.
Thalidomide	Abnormal development of the limbs, e.g., meromelia (partial absence) and amelia (complete absence); facial anomalies; systemic anomalies, e.g., cardiac and kidney defects.
Trimethadione	Developmental delay; V-shaped eyebrows; low-set ears; cleft lip and/or palate.
Valproic acid	Craniofacial anomalies; NTDs; often hydrocephalus; heart and skeletal defects.
Warfarin	Nasal hypoplasia; stippled epiphyses; hypoplastic phalanges; eye anomalies; mental retardation.
CHEMICALS	
Methylmercury	Cerebral atrophy; spasticity; seizures; mental retardation.
PCBs	IUGR; skin discolorization.
INFECTIONS	
Cytomegalovirus	Microcephaly; chorioretinitis; sensorineural loss; delayed psychomotor/mental development; hepatosplenomegaly; hydrocephaly; cerebral palsy; brain (periventricular) calcification.
Herpes simplex virus	Skin vesicles and scarring; chorioretinitis; hepatomegaly; thrombocytopenia; petechiae; hemolytic anemia; hydranencephaly.
Human immunodeficiency virus (HIV)	Growth failure; microcephaly; prominent boxlike forehead; flattened nasal bridge; hypertelorism; triangular philtrum and patulous lips.
Human parvovirus B19	Eye defects; degenerative changes in fetal tissues.
Rubella virus	IUGR; postnatal growth retardation; cardiac and great vessel malformations; microcephaly; sensorineural deafness; cataract; microphthalmos; glaucoma (Fig. 5–12); pigmented retinopathy; mental retardation; newborn bleeding; hepatosplenomegaly; osteopathy.
Toxoplasma gondii	Microcephaly; mental retardation; microphthalmia; hydrocephaly; chorioretinitis; cerebral calcifications.
Treponema pallidum	Hydrocephalus; congenital deafness; mental retardation; abnormal teeth and bones.
Venezuelan equine encephalitis virus	Microcephaly; microphthalmia; cerebral agenesis; CNS necrosis; hydrocephalus.
Varicella virus	Cutaneous scars (dermatome distribution); neurological anomalies (limb paresis, hydrocephaly, seizures, etc.); cataracts; microphthalmia; Horner syndrome; optic atrophy; nystagmus; chorioretinitis; microcephaly; mental retardation; skeletal anomalies (hypoplasia of limbs, fingers, and toes, etc.); urogenital anomalies.
HIGH LEVELS OF IONIZING RADIATION	Microcephaly; mental retardation; skeletal anomalies.

* The spectrum and severity of congenital anomalies may vary from one case to another. For more information see Holmes. 1992; Persaud, 1990; Shepard, 1992, and Moore and Persaud, 1993.
(Adapted from Moore KL and Persaud TVN: *The Developing Human,* ed 5. Philadelphia, WB Saunders, 1993.)

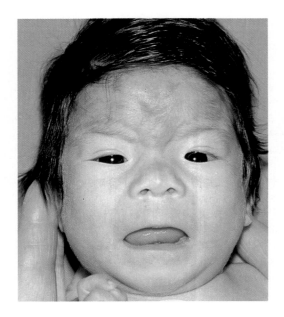

Figure 5–11. Neonate with the fetal alcohol syndrome. Note the thin upper lip, short palpebral fissures, flat nasal bridge, short nose, and elongated and poorly formed philtrum. Maternal alcohol abuse is thought to be the most common environmental cause of mental retardation. (Courtesy of Dr. A.E. Chudley, Professor of Pediatrics and Child Health, Children's Centre, Winnipeg, Manitoba, Canada).

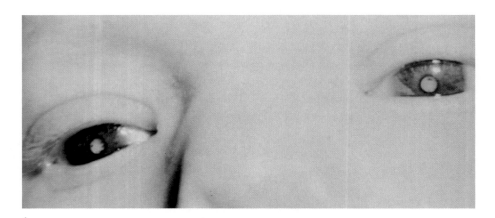

A

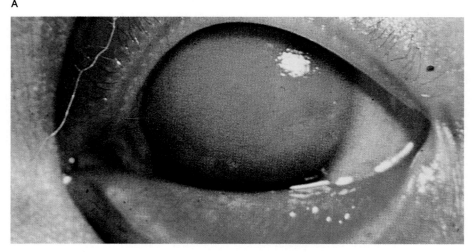

B

Figure 5–12. *A,* Typical bilateral congenital cataracts due to the teratogenic effects of the rubella virus. Cardiac defects and deafness are other common congenital defects. *B,* Severe congenital glaucoma due to rubella. Observe the dense corneal haze, enlarged corneal diameter, and deep anterior chamber. (Part *A* courtesy of Dr. Richard Bargy, Department of Ophthalmology, Cornell-New York Hospital. Part *B* courtesy of Dr. Daniel I. Weiss, Department of Ophthalmology, New York University College of Medicine. From Cooper LA et al.: *Am J Dis Child 110:*416, 1965. Copyright 1965, American Medical Association.)

Radiation as a Teratogen

Exposure to *ionizing radiation* may injure embryonic cells, resulting in cell death, chromosome injury, and retardation of mental development and physical growth. The severity of the embryonic damage is related to the absorbed dose, the dose rate, and the stage of embryonic or fetal development during which the exposure occurs. In the past, large amounts of ionizing radiation (hundreds to several thousand rads) were given inadvertently to embryos and fetuses of pregnant women who had cancer of the cervix. In all cases, their embryos were severely malformed or killed.

There is no proof that human congenital anomalies have been caused by diagnostic levels of radiation. Scattered radiation from an x-ray examination of a part of the body that is not near the uterus (e.g., the chest, sinuses, teeth) produces a dose of only a few millirads, which is not teratogenic to the embryo.

6

EMBRYONIC BODY CAVITIES AND THE DIAPHRAGM

Early development of the intraembryonic coelom (embryonic body cavity) during the third week is described and illustrated in Chapter 2. By the fourth week, the coelom appears as a horseshoe-shaped cavity in the cardiogenic and lateral mesoderm (Fig. 6–1). The curve or bend in this cavity represents the future *pericardial cavity* and its limbs (or lateral parts) indicate the future *pleural and peritoneal cavities.*

The distal part of each limb of the intraembryonic coelom opens into the *extraembryonic coelom* at the lateral edges of the embryonic disc (Fig. 6–1). This communication is important because most of the midgut normally herniates through this communication into the umbilical cord where it develops into most of the small intestine and part of the large intestine. During embryonic folding in the horizontal plane, the limbs of the intraembryonic coelom are brought together on the ventral aspect of the embryo (Fig. 6–2). The ventral mesentery degenerates in the region of the future peritoneal cavity, resulting in a large embryonic peritoneal cavity extending from the heart to the pelvic region (Fig. 6–2F).

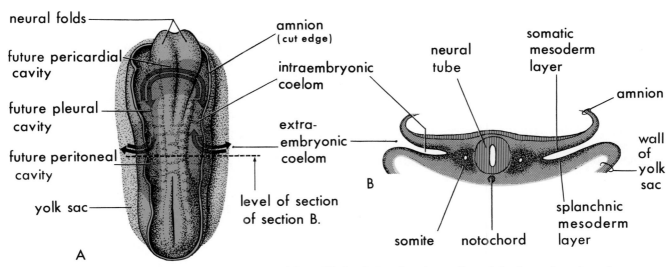

Figure 6–1. *A,* Drawings of an embryo (about 22 days) showing the outline of the horseshoe-shaped intraembryonic coelom. The amnion has been removed and the coelom is shown as if the embryo were translucent. The continuity of the intraembryonic coelom, as well as the communication of its right and left extremities with the extraembryonic coelom, are indicated by arrows. *B,* Transverse section through the embryo at the level shown in *A.* (From Moore KL and Persaud TVN: *The Developing Human,* ed 5. Philadelphia, WB Saunders, 1993.)

THE EMBRYONIC BODY CAVITY

The well-defined intraembryonic coelom gives rise to three well-defined coelomic (body) cavities in the fourth week: (1) a large *pericardial cavity* (Fig. 6–2B), (2) two *pericardioperitoneal canals* connecting the pericardial and peritoneal cavities (Fig. 6–2B), and (3) a large *peritoneal cavity* (Fig. 6–2C to E). These cavities have a parietal wall lined by mesothelium (future parietal peritoneum) derived from the somatic mesoderm, and a visceral wall covered by mesothelium derived from the splanchnic mesoderm (Fig. 6–2E). The peritoneal cavity is connected with the extraembryonic coelom but is separated from it during the tenth week as the intestines return to the abdomen from the umbilical cord (see Fig. 9–2).

During formation of the *head fold* during the fifth week, the heart and pericardial cavity are carried ventrocaudally, anterior to the foregut (Figs. 6–2A). As a result, the pericardial cavity opens dorsally into the pericardioperitoneal canals on each side of the foregut (Fig. 6–2B). After embryonic folding, the caudal part of the foregut, the midgut, and hindgut are suspended in the peritoneal cavity from the posterior abdominal wall by the **dorsal mesentery** (Fig. 6–2D).

A mesentery is a double layer of peritoneum. Transiently, the dorsal and ventral mesenteries divide the peritoneal cavity into right and left halves, but the ventral mesentery soon disappears, except where it is attached to the caudal part of the foregut (primordium of the stomach and the proximal part of the duodenum). The peritoneal cavity then becomes a continuous space (Fig. 6–2E). The arteries supplying the primitive gut, (i.e., the celiac [foregut], the superior mesenteric [midgut], and the inferior mesenteric [hindgut]), pass from the dorsal aorta between the layers of the dorsal mesentery.

Division of the Embryonic Body Cavity

Each pericardioperitoneal canal lies lateral to the foregut (future esophagus) and dorsal to the *septum transversum,* which is part of the future diaphragm (Fig. 6–2A and 6–3). Partitions form concurrently in each pericardioperitoneal canal which soon separate the pericardial cavity from the pleural cavities and the pleural cavities from the peritoneal cavity. Due to *growth of the bronchial buds* (primordia of the lungs) into the pericardioperitoneal canals, a pair of membranous ridges is produced in the lateral wall of each canal. The cranial ridges, called *pleuropericardial membranes,* are located superior to the developing lungs and the caudal ridges, called *pleuroperitoneal membranes,* are located inferior to them.

THE PLEUROPERICARDIAL MEMBRANES (Fig. 6–3B). As these cranial ridges enlarge, they form partitions that separate the pericardial cavity from the pleural cavities. At this stage, the *bronchial buds* are small relative to the heart and pericardial cavity. They grow laterally from the caudal end of the trachea into the corresponding pericardioperitoneal canal (pleural canal), which becomes the *primitive pleural cavity.* As these cavities expand ventrally around the heart, they extend into the body wall and split the mesenchyme into (1) an outer layer that becomes the thoracic wall and (2) an inner layer (the pleuropericardial membrane) that becomes the *fibrous pericardium,* the outer fibrous layer of the pericardial sac.

THE PLEUROPERITONEAL MEMBRANES. As these caudal partitions in the pericardioperitoneal canals enlarge, they gradually separate the pleural cavities from the peritoneal cavity. This pair of membranes is produced as the developing lungs and pleural cavities expand and invade the body wall. They are attached dorsolaterally to the abdominal wall and their crescentic free edges initially project into the caudal ends of the pericardioperitoneal canals. They become relatively more prominent as the lungs enlarge and the liver expands.

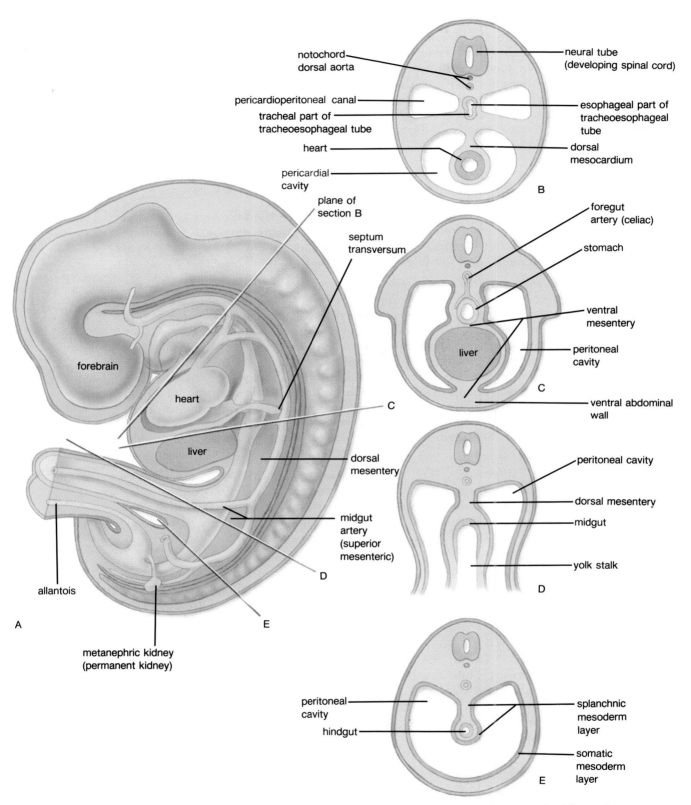

Figure 6-2. Drawings illustrating the body cavities and mesenteries at the beginning of the fifth week. *A,* Schematic longitudinal section. Note that the dorsal mesentery serves as a pathway for the arteries supplying the developing gut (e.g., midgut artery). Nerves and lymphatics also pass between the layers of this mesentery. *B* to *E,* Transverse sections through the embryo at the levels indicated in *A.* The ventral mesentery disappears, except in the region of the terminal esophagus, stomach, and the first part of the duodenum. Note that the right and left parts of the peritoneal cavity, which are separate in *C,* are continuous in *E.*

During the sixth week, the pleuroperitoneal membranes extend ventromedially until their free edges fuse with the dorsal mesentery of the esophagus and the septum transversum (Fig. 6–3C). This separates the pleural cavities from the peritoneal cavity. *Closure of the pleuroperitoneal openings* is assisted by the migration of myoblasts (primitive muscle cells) into the pleuroperitoneal membranes, which form posterolateral parts of the diaphragm (Fig. 6–3E). The pleuroperitoneal opening on the right side closes slightly before the left one. The reason for this is uncertain, but it may be related to the relatively large right lobe of the liver at this stage of development.

DEVELOPMENT OF THE DIAPHRAGM

This dome-shaped, musculotendinous partition separates the thoracic and abdominal cavities. It has a complex embryonic origin. *The diaphragm develops from four structures:* the septum transversum, the pleuroperitoneal membranes, the dorsal mesentery of the esophagus, and the lateral body walls (Fig. 6–3).

THE SEPTUM TRANSVERSUM. This transverse septum, composed of mesoderm, is the primordium of the *central tendon of the diaphragm* (Fig. 6–3E). It is located caudal to the pericardial cavity and partially separates it from the developing peritoneal cavity. The septum transversum is first identifiable at the end of the third week as a mass of mesodermal tissue cranial to the pericardial cavity. After the head folds ventrally during the fourth week, the septum transversum forms a thick incomplete partition, or partial diaphragm, between the pericardial and abdominal cavities (Fig. 6–3B). The septum transversum does not separate the thoracic and abdominal cavities completely. It leaves a large opening, the *pericardioperitoneal canal,* on each side of the esophagus. The septum transversum fuses with the mesenchyme ventral to the esophagus (primordial mediastinum) and with the pleuroperitoneal membranes (Fig. 6–3C).

THE PLEUROPERITONEAL MEMBRANES (Fig. 6–3C). These membranes fuse with the dorsal mesentery of the esophagus and the septum transversum. This completes the partition between the thoracic and abdominal cavities and forms the *primitive diaphragm.* Although the pleuroperitoneal membranes form large portions of the embryonic diaphragm, they represent relatively small portions of the infant's diaphragm (Fig. 6–3E).

THE DORSAL MESENTERY OF THE ESOPHAGUS. As previously described, the septum transversum and pleuroperitoneal membranes fuse with the dorsal mesentery of the esophagus. This mesentery constitutes the median portion of the diaphragm. The *crura of the diaphragm* develop from myoblasts that grow into the dorsal mesentery of the esophagus (Fig. 6–3E).

THE LATERAL BODY WALLS. During the ninth to twelfth weeks the lungs and pleural cavities enlarge, "burrowing" into the lateral body walls. During this "excavation" process the tissue is split into two layers: (1) an outer layer that becomes part of the definitive abdominal wall, and (2) an inner layer that contributes muscle to peripheral portions of the diaphragm, external to the parts derived from the pleuroperitoneal membranes (Fig. 6–3E).

Congenital Diaphragmatic Defects

Despite the rather complex embryologic development of the diaphragm, congenital anomalies of it are relatively uncommon.

CONGENITAL DIAPHRAGMATIC HERNIA (CDH). *Posterolateral defect of the diaphragm* is the only relatively common congenital abnormality of the diaphragm (Figs. 6–4 and 6–5). It occurs about once in 2200 newborn infants (Harrison, 1991) and is

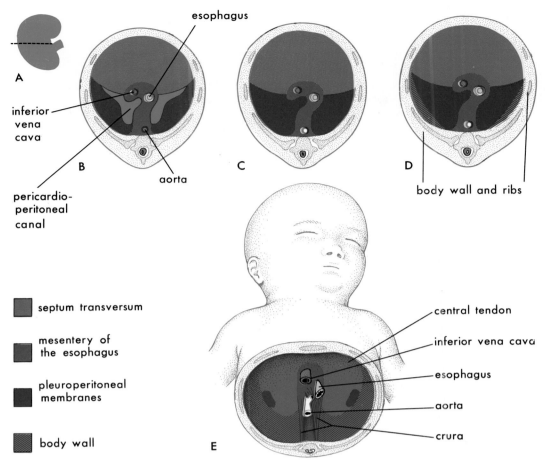

esophagus

inferior
vena
cava

pericardio-
peritoneal
canal

aorta

A

B

C

D

body wall and ribs

■ septum transversum

▨ mesentery of
the esophagus

■ pleuroperitoneal
membranes

▨ body wall

E

central tendon

inferior vena cava

esophagus

aorta

crura

Figure 6–3. Drawings illustrating development of the diaphragm as viewed from below. *A*, Sketch of a lateral view of an embryo at the end of the fifth week (actual size), indicating the level of sections below it. *B*, Transverse section showing the unfused pleuroperitoneal membranes and pericardioperitoneal canals. *C*, Similar section at the end of the sixth week after fusion of the pleuroperitoneal membranes with the other two diaphragmatic components. *D*, Transverse section of a 12-week embryo after ingrowth of the fourth diaphragmatic component from the body wall. *E*, View of the diaphragm of a neonate indicating the embryological origin of its components. (From Moore KL and Persaud TVN: *The Developing Human,* ed 5. Philadelphia, WB Saunders, 1993.)

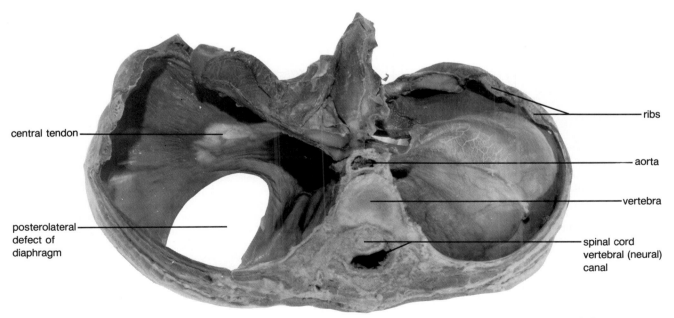

central tendon

posterolateral
defect of
diaphragm

ribs

aorta

vertebra

spinal cord
vertebral (neural)
canal

Figure 6–4. Photograph of a transverse section through the thoracic region of a stillborn infant, viewed from the thorax. Note the large, left posterolateral defect in the diaphragm, which permitted the abdominal contents to pass into the thorax (CDH), as shown in Figure 6–5*A*.

congenital diaphragmatic hernia

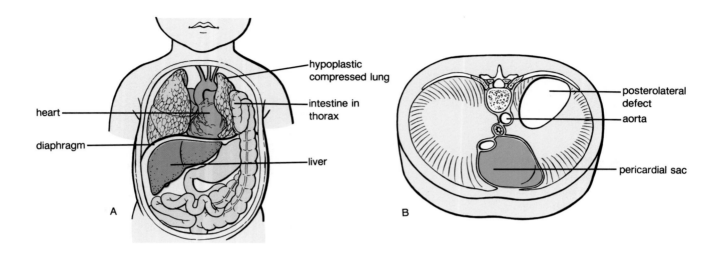

eventration of the diaphragm

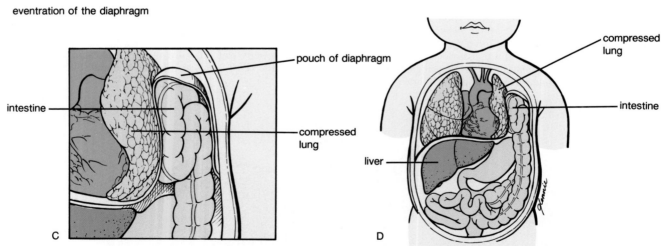

Figure 6–5.   *A,* "Windows" have been drawn on the thorax and abdomen to show the herniation of the intestine into the thorax through a posterolateral defect in the left side of the diaphragm similar to that illustrated in Figure 6–4. Note that the left lung is compressed and hypoplastic. Posterolateral defects of the diaphragm usually occur on the left side (75 to 90 per cent). *B,* Drawing of a diaphragm with a large posterolateral defect on the left side due to abnormal formation and/or fusion of the pleuroperitonal membrane on the left side with the mesoesophagus and the septum transversum. *C* and *D,* Eventration of the diaphragm due to defective muscular development of the diaphragm. The abdominal viscera are displaced into the thorax within a pouch of diaphragmatic tissue.

associated with CHD (herniation of abdominal contents into the thoracic cavity) and life-threatening breathing difficulties. *Polyhydramnios* is usually present also. *Prenatal diagnosis of CDH* depends on the sonographic demonstration of abdominal organs in the thorax.

CDH, usually unilateral (97 per cent) results from defective formation and/or fusion of the pleuroperitoneal membrane with the other three parts of the diaphragm (Fig. 6–3). The defect commonly consists of a large opening[1] in the posterolateral region of the diaphragm (Figs. 6–4 and 6–5). The defect usually occurs on the left side (75 to 90 per cent); this preponderance is likely related to the earlier closure of the right pleuroperitoneal opening.

The pleuroperitoneal membranes normally fuse with the other three diaphragmatic components by the end of the sixth week (Fig. 6–3C). If a pleuroperitoneal membrane is unfused when the intestines return to the abdomen from the umbilical cord in the tenth week, the intestine may pass into the thorax. Often the stomach, spleen, and most of the intestines herniate. Uncommonly, the liver and a kidney also pass into the thoracic cavity and displace the lungs and heart. The viscera usually can move freely through the defect; consequently, they may be in the thoracic cavity when the infant is lying down and in the abdominal cavity when the infant is upright. Most infants born with CDH die not because there is a defect in the diaphragm or viscera in the chest, but because the lungs are hypoplastic due to compression during their development (Harrison, 1991).

The lungs in infants with CDH are often hypoplastic and greatly reduced in size. The growth retardation results from lack of room for them to develop normally. The lungs are often aerated and achieve their normal size after reduction (repositioning) of the herniated viscera and repair of the defect in the diaphragm; but the mortality rate is high, approximately 76 per cent. If necessary, CDH can be diagnosed and repaired prenatally between 22 and 28 weeks of gestation, but this intervention carries considerable risk to the fetus and mother (Harrison, 1991).

[1] Sometimes referred to clinically as the foramen of Bochdalek.

7

THE BRANCHIAL OR
PHARYNGEAL APPARATUS

During the fourth and fifth weeks, the primordial pharynx is bounded laterally by barlike *branchial or pharyngeal arches* (Figs. 7–1 and 7–2). Each arch consists of a core of mesenchyme covered externally by ectoderm and internally by endoderm. The original mesenchyme in each arch is derived from intraembryonic mesoderm. Later, *neural crest cells* migrate into the arches and are the major source of connective tissue components, including cartilage, bone, and ligaments, in the oral and facial regions. Each arch also contains an artery, a cartilage rod, a nerve, and a muscular component.

Externally, the arches are separated by *branchial or pharyngeal grooves* (Figs. 7–1 and 7–2). Internally, the arches are separated by evaginations of the pharynx called *pharyngeal pouches.* Where the ectoderm of a groove contacts the endoderm of a pouch, *branchial or pharyngeal membranes* are formed. The pouches, arches, grooves, and membranes make up the branchial or pharyngeal apparatus. Development of the tongue, face, lips, jaws, palate, pharynx, and neck largely involves transformation of the branchial or pharyngeal apparatus into adult structures (Figs. 7–3 to 7–8). The adult derivatives of the various arch components are summarized in Table 7–1.

The branchial or pharyngeal grooves disappear except for the first pair, which persists as the *external acoustic meatus* (Fig. 7–9). The branchial or pharyngeal membranes also disappear except for the first pair, which becomes the *tympanic membranes.* The first pharyngeal pouch gives rise to the *tympanic cavity,* mastoid antrum, and auditory tube. The second pharyngeal pouch is associated with the development of the *palatine tonsil.* The *thymus* is derived from the third pair of pharyngeal pouches, and the *parathyroid glands* are formed from the third and fourth pairs of pharyngeal pouches (Fig. 7–6).

The *thyroid gland* develops from a downgrowth from the floor of the primordial pharynx in the region where the tongue develops (Figs. 7–5 and 7–6). The parafollicular cells (C cells) in the thyroid gland are derived from the *ultimobranchial bodies,* which are derived mainly from the fourth pair of pharyngeal pouches.

The face develops from five primordia: the single frontonasal prominence and the paired maxillary and mandibular prominences (Figs. 7–9 to 7–11). The *palate* develops from two primordia, the primary palate (median palatine process) and the secondary palate (Figs. 7–12 and 7–18). The secondary palate develops from two mesenchymal projections that extend from the internal aspects of the maxillary prominences. These shelflike structures are called lateral palatine processes or palatal shelves. Anteriorly, these processes (shelves) fuse with the primary palate and later with each other.

Most congenital anomalies of the head and neck originate during transformation of the branchial apparatus into adult structures. Branchial cysts, sinuses, and fistulas

Text continued on page 132

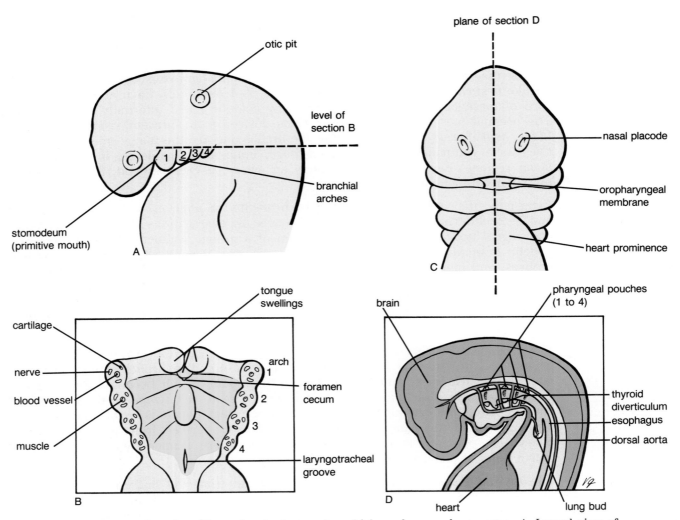

Figure 7–1. Drawings illustrating the human branchial or pharyngeal apparatus. *A,* Lateral view of the cranial part of an early embryo. *B,* Horizontal section through the cranial region of the embryo. *C,* Ventral or facial view illustrating the relationship of the first arch to the stomodeum. At this stage the oropharyngeal membrane separates the stomodeum from the primitive pharynx. *D,* Schematic drawing showing the pharyngeal pouches and the related arteries known as aortic arches.

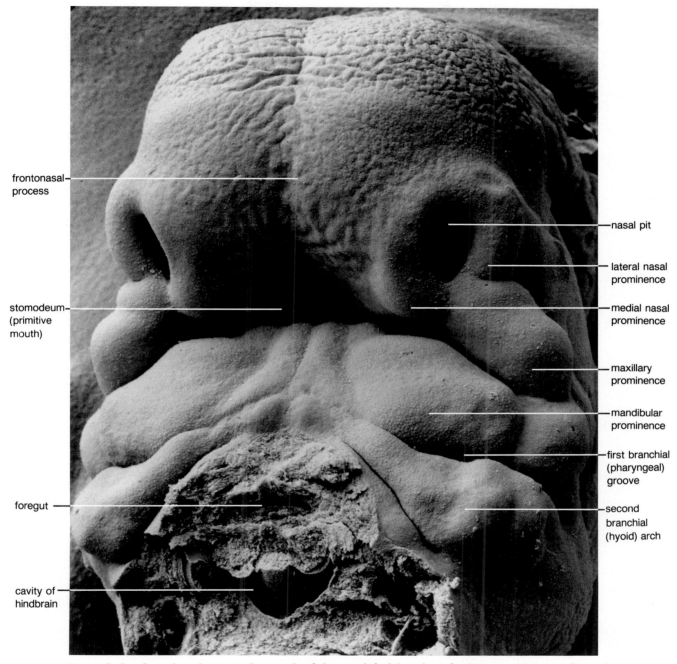

frontonasal process

stomodeum (primitive mouth)

foregut

cavity of hindbrain

nasal pit

lateral nasal prominence

medial nasal prominence

maxillary prominence

mandibular prominence

first branchial (pharyngeal) groove

second branchial (hyoid) arch

Figure 7–2.   Scanning electron micrograph of the craniofacial region of a human embryo at Carnegie stage 16, about 37 days (CRL 10.5 mm). The wide stomodeum (primordial mouth) is limited caudally by the fused mandibular prominences. The nasal pits are surrounded by the medial and lateral nasal prominences and the maxillary prominences. At this stage, the medial nasal prominences have not merged but the mandibular prominences have fused. (Courtesy of Professor Dr. Klaus Hinrichsen, Ruhr-Universitat, Bochum, Germany.)

TABLE 7-1.   STRUCTURES DERIVED FROM BRANCHIAL OR PHARYNGEAL ARCH COMPONENTS

Arch	Nerve	Muscles	Skeletal Structures	Ligaments
First (mandibular)	Trigeminal (V)	Muscles of mastication	Malleus	Anterior ligament of malleus
		Mylohyoid and anterior belly of digastric	Incus	Sphenomandibular ligament
		Tensor tympani		
		Tensor veli palatini		
Second (hyoid)	Facial (VII)	Muscles of facial expressions	Stapes	Stylohyoid ligament
		Stapedius	Styloid process	
		Stylohyoid	Lesser cornu of hyoid bone	
		Posterior belly of digastric	Upper part of body of the hyoid bone	
Third	Glossopharyngeal (IX)	Stylopharyngeus	Greater cornu of hyoid bone	
			Lower part of body of the hyoid bone	
Fourth and Sixth	Superior laryngeal branch of vagus (X)	Cricothyroid	Thyroid cartilage	
		Levator veli palatini	Cricoid cartilage	
	Recurrent laryngeal branch of vagus (X)	Constrictors of pharynx	Arytenoid cartilage	
		Intrinsic muscles of larynx	Corniculate cartilage	
		Striated muscles of the esophagus	Cuneiform cartilage	

(Adapted from Moore KL, Persaud TVN: *The Developing Human,* ed 5. Philadelphia, WB Saunders, 1993.)

may develop from parts of the second branchial groove, the cervical sinus, or the second pharyngeal pouch that fail to obliterate. An *ectopic thyroid gland* results when the thyroid gland fails to descend completely from its site of origin in the tongue (Fig. 7–5). The thyroglossal duct may persist or remnants of it may give rise to a *thyroglossal duct cyst* (Fig. 7–7). Infected cysts may perforate the skin and form *thyroglossal duct sinuses* that open anteriorly in the median plane of the neck.

Due to the complex development of the face and palate, congenital anomalies of the face and palate are common. *Anomalies usually result from maldevelopment of neural crest tissue* that gives rise to the skeletal and connective tissue primordia of the face. Neural crest cells may be deficient in number, may not complete their migration to the face, or they may fail in their inductive capacity (Sperber, 1989). Anomalies of the face and palate result from an arrest of development and/or a failure of fusion of the prominences and processes involved.

Cleft lip is a common congenital anomaly (Figs. 7–13 to 7–17). Although it is frequently associated with cleft palate, cleft lip and palate are etiologically distinct anomalies that involve different developmental processes occurring at different times. Cleft lip results from failure of mesenchymal masses in the medial nasal and the maxillary prominences to merge, whereas *cleft palate* results from failure of mesenchymal masses in the palatine processes (palatal shelves) to meet and fuse.

Most cases of cleft lip, with or without cleft palate, are caused by a combination of genetic and environmental factors *(multifactorial inheritance)*. These factors interfere with the migration of neural crest cells into the maxillary prominences of the first branchial and pharyngeal arch. If the number of cells is insufficient, clefting of the lip and/or palate may occur. Other cellular and molecular mechanisms may be involved (Ferguson, 1988; Hall, 1988; Greene, 1989; Sperber, 1989).

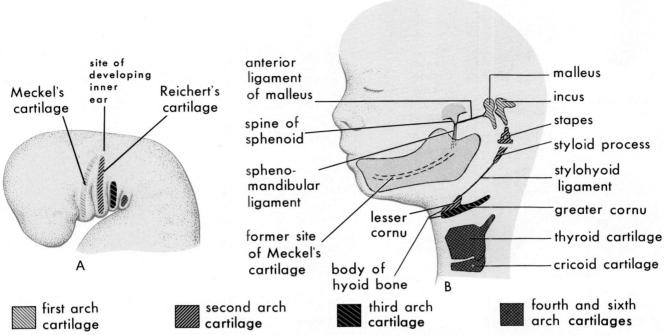

Figure 7–3. *A*, Schematic lateral view of the head and neck region of a 4-week embryo showing the location of the cartilages in the branchial or pharyngeal arches. *B*, Similar view of a 24-week fetus illustrating the adult derivatives of the arch cartilages. Note that the mandible is formed by membranous ossification of mesenchymal tissue surrounding Meckel's cartilage. (From Moore KL and Persaud TVN: *The Developing Human*, ed 5. Philadelphia, WB Saunders, 1993.)

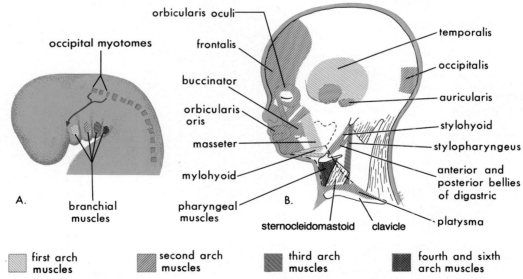

Figure 7–4. *A*, Sketch of lateral view of the head and neck region of a 4-week embryo showing the branchial or pharyngeal muscles. The *arrow* shows the pathway taken by myoblasts (developing muscle cells) from the occipital myotomes to form the tongue musculature. *B*, Sketch of the head and neck of a 20-week fetus dissected to show the muscles derived from the branchial or pharyngeal arches. Parts of the platysma and sternocleidomastoid muscles have been removed to show the deeper muscles. Note that myoblasts from the second branchial arch migrate from the neck region to the head and give rise to the muscles of facial expression. These muscles are therefore supplied by the facial nerve, the nerve of the second arch. (From Moore KL and Persaud TVN: *The Developing Human*, ed 5. Philadelphia, WB Saunders, 1993.)

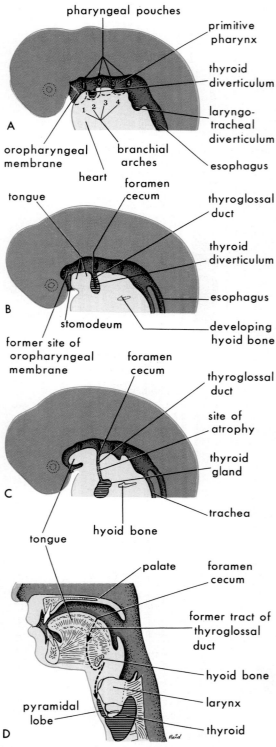

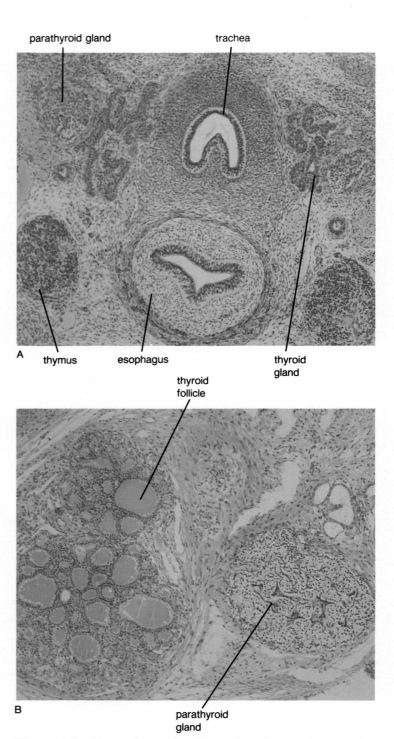

Figure 7–5. *A*, *B*, and *C*, Schematic sagittal sections of the head and neck region of embryos at four, five, and six weeks, respectively, illustrating successive stages of development of the thyroid gland. *D*, Similar section of an adult head, showing the path taken by the thyroid gland during its descent, as indicated by the former tract of the thyroglossal duct. (From Moore KL and Persaud TVN: *The Developing Human*, ed 5. Philadelphia, WB Saunders, 1993.)

Figure 7–6. Photomicrographs illustrating the histology of the thyroid and parathyroid glands (×60). *A*, Thyroid and parathyroid glands located lateral to the trachea. The lobes of the developing thymus are located lateral to the esophagus. *B*, The thyroid and parathyroid glands at 21 weeks (×130). Colloid is first visible in the follicles at 11 weeks; thyroxine forms shortly thereafter.

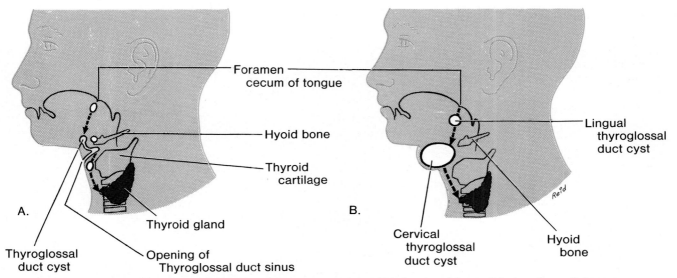

Foramen cecum of tongue

Hyoid bone

Thyroid cartilage

Thyroid gland

A.

Thyroglossal duct cyst

Opening of Thyroglossal duct sinus

B.

Lingual thyroglossal duct cyst

Cervical thyroglossal duct cyst

Hyoid bone

Figure 7–7. *A,* Diagrammatic sketch of the head and neck showing the possible locations of thyroglossal duct cysts. A thyroglossal duct sinus is also illustrated. The *broken line* indicates the course taken by the thyroglossal duct during descent of the developing thyroid gland from the foramen cecum in the tongue to its final position in the anterior part of the neck. *B,* Similar sketch illustrating lingual and cervical thyroglossal duct cysts. Most thyroglossal duct cysts are located just inferior to the hyoid bone. (From Moore KL and Persaud TVN: *The Developing Human,* ed 5. Philadelphia, WB Saunders, 1993.)

Figure 7–8. Typical thyroglossal duct cyst in a female child. The round, firm mass (indicated by the sketch) produced a swelling in the median plane of the neck just inferior to the hyoid bone.

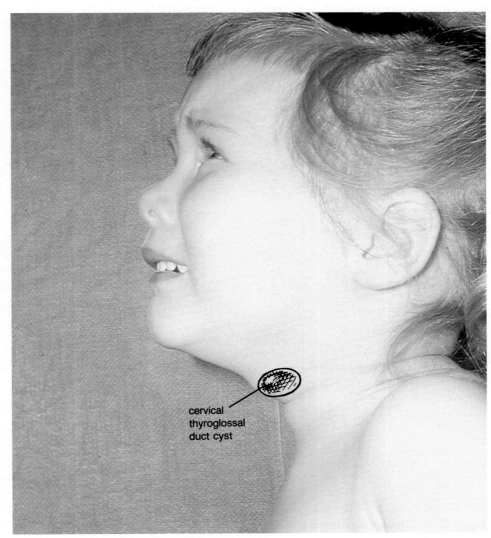

cervical thyroglossal duct cyst

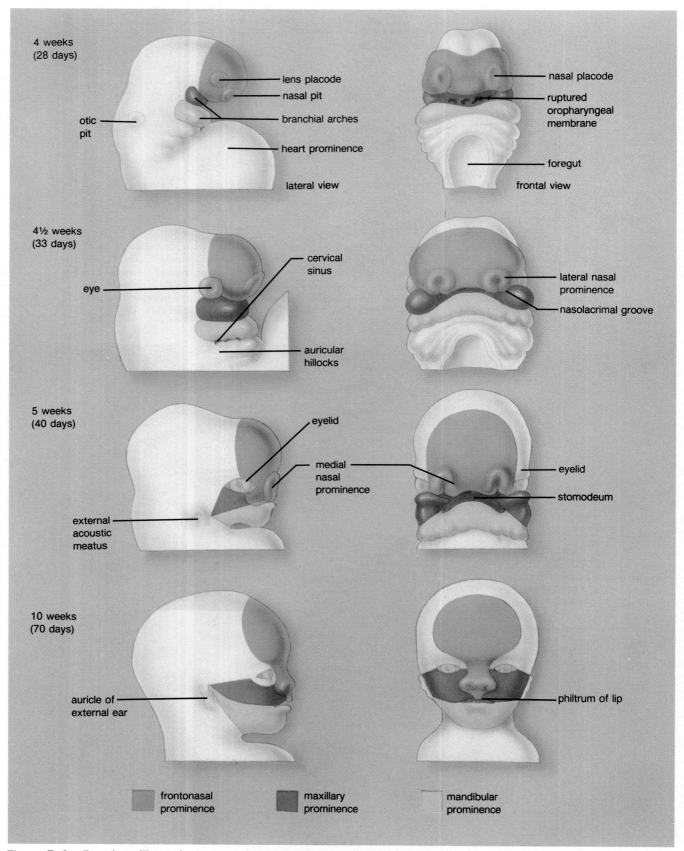

Figure 7–9. Drawings illustrating progressive stages in the development of the face from the fourth to tenth weeks. Observe that the face develops from five primordia that surround the stomodeum (primordium of mouth). The prominences are a single frontonasal prominence and paired maxillary and mandibular prominences.

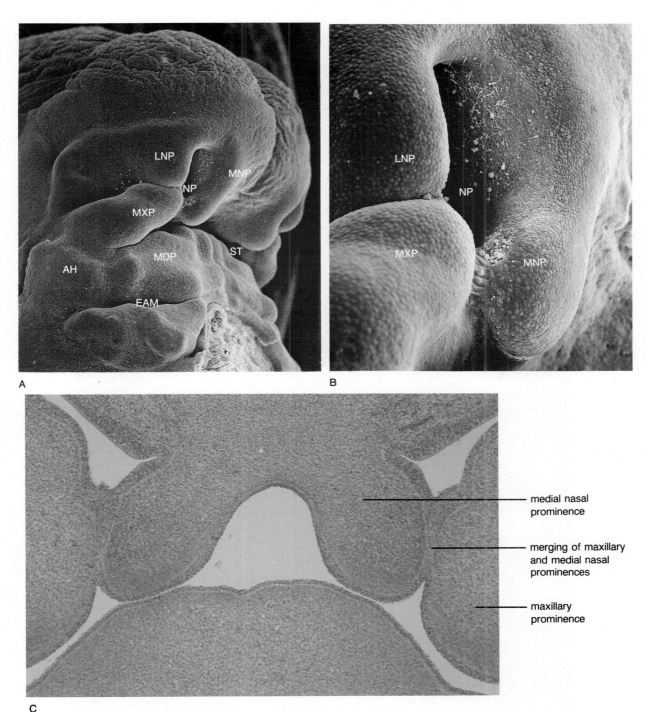

Figure 7–10. *A,* Scanning electron micrograph of the craniofacial region of a human embryo at Carnegie stage 16, about 41 days (CRL 10.8 mm), viewed obliquely. The maxillary prominence (MXP) appears puffed up laterally and is wedged between the lateral (LNP) and medial (MNP) nasal prominences surrounding the nasal pit (NP). The auricular hillocks (AH) can be seen on both sides of the groove between the first two arches which will form the external acoustic meatus (EAM). *B,* Scanning electron micrograph of the right nasal region of a human embryo of about 41 days showing the maxillary and nasal prominences. Epithelial bridges can be seen between these prominences. Observe the furrow representing the nasolacrimal groove between the maxillary prominence (MXP) and the lateral nasal prominence (LNP). Observe the large nasal pit (NP). *C,* Photomicrograph of a coronal section of the face of an embryo at Carnegie stage 18, about 44 days, showing the medial nasal prominences fusing with the maxillary prominences (×25). (Parts *A* and *B* are from Hinrichsen K: *The early development of morphology and patterns of the face in the human embryo.* In *Advances in Anatomy, Embryology, and Cell Biology.* Vol. 98. New York, Springer-Verlag, 1985).

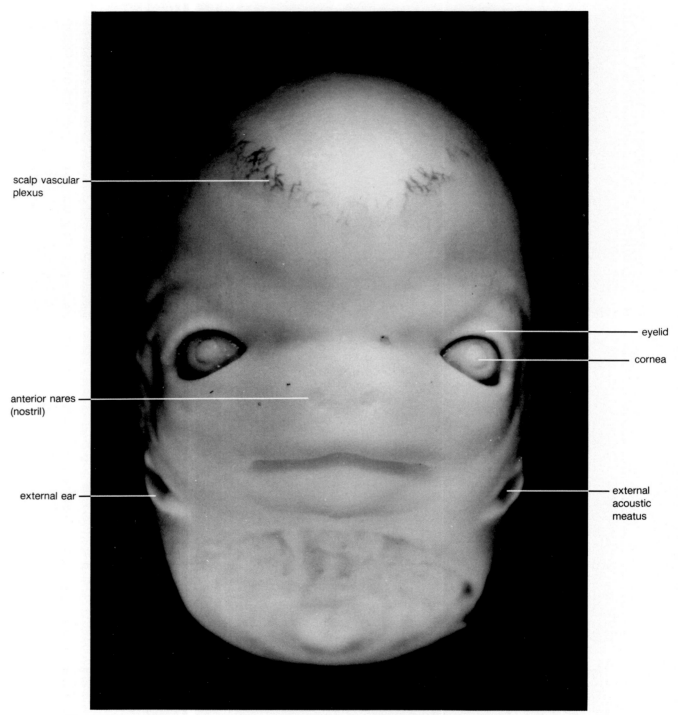

Figure 7–11. Ventral view of the face of an embryo at Carnegie stage 22, about 54 days (×15). For the appearance and size of an embryo at this stage, see Fig. 2–24. Observe that the eyes are widely separated and the ears low-set at this stage. (From Nishimura H et al: *Prenatal Development of the Human with Special Reference to Craniofacial Structures: An Atlas.* U.S. Department of Health, Education, and Welfare, NIH, Bethesda, 1977).

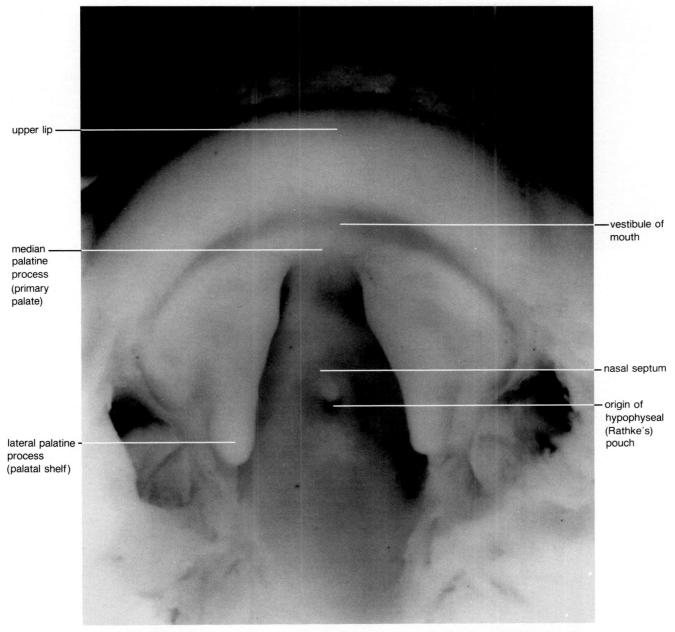

Figure 7-12. Roof of the oral cavity of an embryo at Carnegie stage 22, about 54 days (×20). Note that the lateral palatine processes (palatal shelves) are widely separated at this stage. They fuse in the median plane with each other and the nasal septum at twelve weeks. Failure of these processes to fuse, as shown in (Fig. 7-18) results in various types of cleft palate. (From Nishimura H et al: *Prenatal Development of the Human with Special Reference to Craniofacial Structures: An Atlas.* U.S. Department of Health, Education, and Welfare, NIH, Bethesda, 1977).

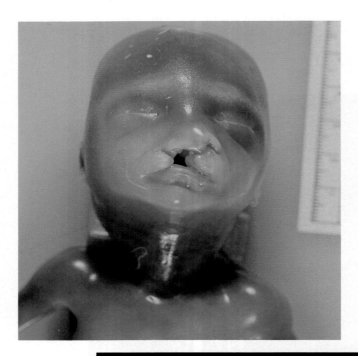

Figure 7-13. Male fetus (16 weeks) with unilateral cleft lip and palate. The eyelids are normally fused at this age. They open during the twenty-sixth week. (Courtesy of Dr. D.K. Kalousek, Professor, Department of Pathology, University of British Columbia, Vancouver, B.C., Canada.)

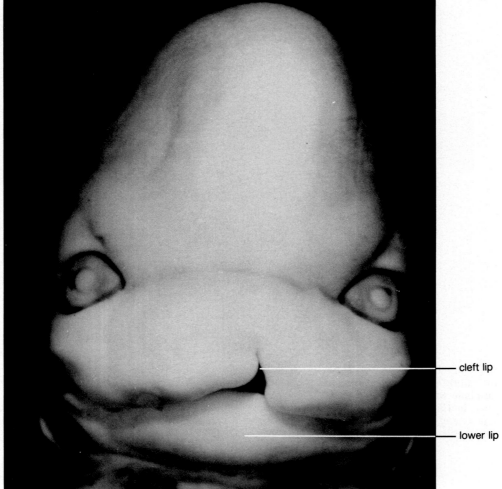

cleft lip

lower lip

Figure 7-14. Ventral view of the face of an embryo at Carnegie stage 20 (about 51 days) with a unilateral cleft lip. (From Nishimura H et al: *Prenatal Development of the Human with Special Reference to Craniofacial Structures: An Atlas.* U.S. Department of Health, Education, and Welfare, NIH, Bethesda, 1977).

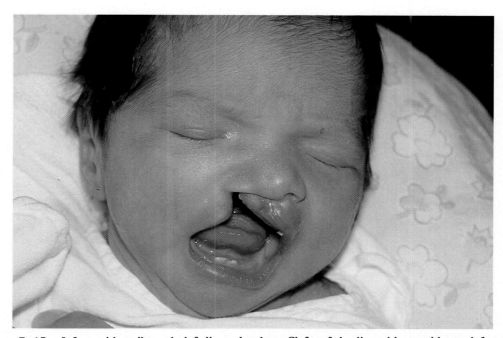

Figure 7-15. Infant with unilateral cleft lip and palate. Clefts of the lip, with or without cleft palate, occur about once in 1000 births; 60 to 80 per cent of affected infants are males. Unilateral cleft lip results from failure of the maxillary prominence on the affected side to unite with the merged medial nasal prominences (Figs. 7-9 and 7-10). (Courtesy of Dr. A.E. Chudley, Professor of Pediatrics and Child Health, Children's Centre, Winnipeg, Manitoba, Canada).

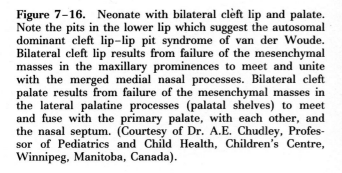

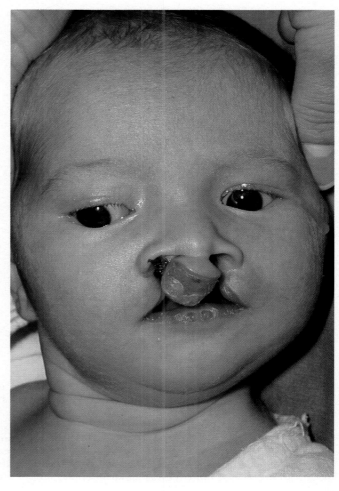

Figure 7-16. Neonate with bilateral cleft lip and palate. Note the pits in the lower lip which suggest the autosomal dominant cleft lip-lip pit syndrome of van der Woude. Bilateral cleft lip results from failure of the mesenchymal masses in the maxillary prominences to meet and unite with the merged medial nasal processes. Bilateral cleft palate results from failure of the mesenchymal masses in the lateral palatine processes (palatal shelves) to meet and fuse with the primary palate, with each other, and the nasal septum. (Courtesy of Dr. A.E. Chudley, Professor of Pediatrics and Child Health, Children's Centre, Winnipeg, Manitoba, Canada).

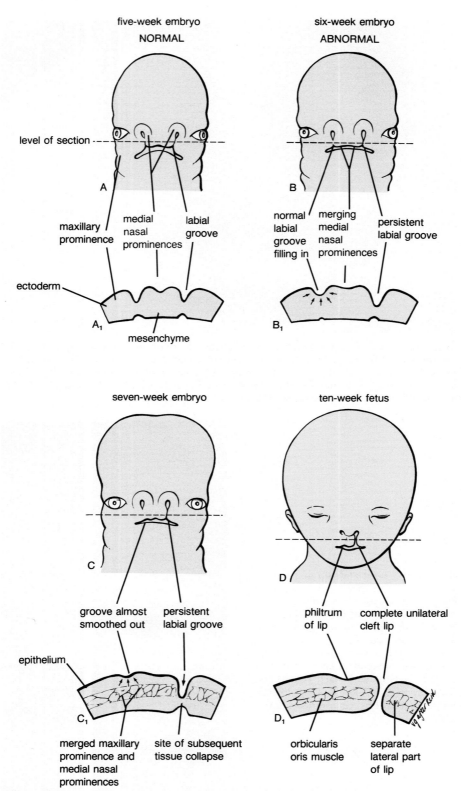

Figure 7–17. Drawings illustrating the embryologic basis of complete unilateral cleft lip. *A,* Five-week embryo. *A₁,* Horizontal section through the head illustrating the grooves between the maxillary prominences and the merging medial nasal prominences. *B,* Six-week embryo showing a persistent labial groove on the left side. *B₁,* Horizontal section through the head showing the groove gradually filling in on the right side following proliferation of mesenchyme *(arrows). C,* Seven-week embryo. *C₁,* Horizontal section through the head showing that the epithelium on the right has almost been pushed out of the groove between the maxillary prominence and medial nasal prominence. *D,* Ten-week fetus with a complete unilateral cleft lip. *D₁,* Horizontal section through the head after stretching of the epithelium and breakdown of the tissues in the floor of the persistent labial groove on the left side forming a complete unilateral cleft lip.

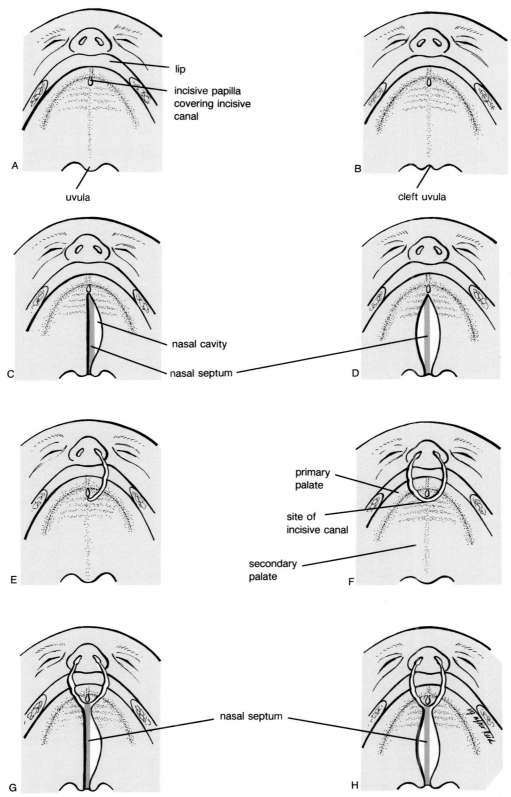

Figure 7–18. Drawings illustrating various types of cleft lip and palate. *A*, Normal lip and palate. *B*, Cleft uvula. *C*, Unilateral cleft of the posterior or secondary palate. *D*, Bilateral cleft of the posterior palate. *E*, Complete unilateral cleft of the lip and alveolar process of the maxilla with a unilateral cleft of the anterior or primary palate. *F*, Complete bilateral cleft of the lip and alveolar processes of the maxillae with bilateral cleft of the anterior palate. *G*, Complete bilateral cleft of the lip and alveolar processes of the maxillae with bilateral cleft of the anterior palate and unilateral cleft of the posterior palate. *H*, Complete bilateral cleft of the lip and alveolar processes of the maxillae with complete bilateral cleft of the anterior and posterior palate.

8

THE RESPIRATORY SYSTEM

The lower respiratory system begins to develop around the middle of the fourth week from a median *laryngotracheal groove* in the floor of the primordial pharynx (see Fig. 7–1*B*). This groove deepens to produce a *laryngotracheal diverticulum,* which soon separates from the foregut as tracheoesophageal folds form and fuse to form the *tracheoesophageal septum* (Figs. 8–1 and 8–2). This results in the formation of the primordial esophagus and the *laryngotracheal tube.* The endoderm of this tube gives rise to the epithelium of the lower respiratory organs and to the *tracheobronchial glands.* The splanchnic mesenchyme surrounding the laryngotracheal tube forms the connective tissue, cartilage, muscle, and blood and lymphatic vessels of these organs (Fig. 8–3).

Branchial or pharyngeal arch mesenchyme contributes to formation of the epiglottis and the connective tissue of the larynx. The laryngeal muscles and the skeleton of the larynx are derived from mesenchyme in the caudal branchial or pharyngeal arches (Fig. 8–1). The cartilages are derived from neural crest cells. The laryngeal cartilages develop from the cartilaginous bars in the fourth and sixth pairs of branchial or pharyngeal arches (Fig. 8–3; also see Table 7–1).

During the fourth week, the laryngotracheal tube develops a *lung bud* at its distal end, which soon divides into two *bronchial buds* during the early part of the fifth week (Fig. 8–1*B*). Each bud soon enlarges to form a *primary bronchus,* and then each of these gives rise to two new bronchial buds, which develop into *secondary bronchi.* The right inferior secondary bronchus soon divides into two bronchi. The secondary bronchi supply the lobes of the developing lungs (Fig. 8–1*C*). Each secondary bronchus undergoes progressive branching to form *segmental bronchi.* Each segmental bronchus with its surrounding mesenchyme is the primordium of a *bronchopulmonary segment.* Branching continues until about 17 orders of branches have formed. Additional airways are formed after birth until about 24 orders of branches are present.

Congenital anomalies of the lower respiratory system are uncommon except for *tracheoesophageal fistula,* which is usually associated with *esophageal atresia* (Fig. 8–4). These anomalies result from faulty partitioning of the foregut into the esophagus and trachea during the fourth and fifth weeks.

Lung development is divided into four stages (Figs. 8–5 and 8–6). During the *pseudoglandular period* (5 to 17 weeks), the bronchi and terminal bronchioles form. During the *canalicular period* (16 to 25 weeks), the lumina of the bronchi and terminal bronchioles enlarge, the respiratory bronchioles and alveolar ducts develop, and the lung tissue becomes highly vascular. During the *terminal sac period* (24 weeks to birth), the alveolar ducts give rise to terminal sacs (or primitive alveoli). The terminal sacs are initially lined with cuboidal epithelium that begins to attenuate to squamous epithelium at about 26 weeks. By this time, capillary networks have proliferated close to the alveolar epithelium, and the lungs are usually sufficiently well-developed to permit survival of the fetus if it is born prematurely.

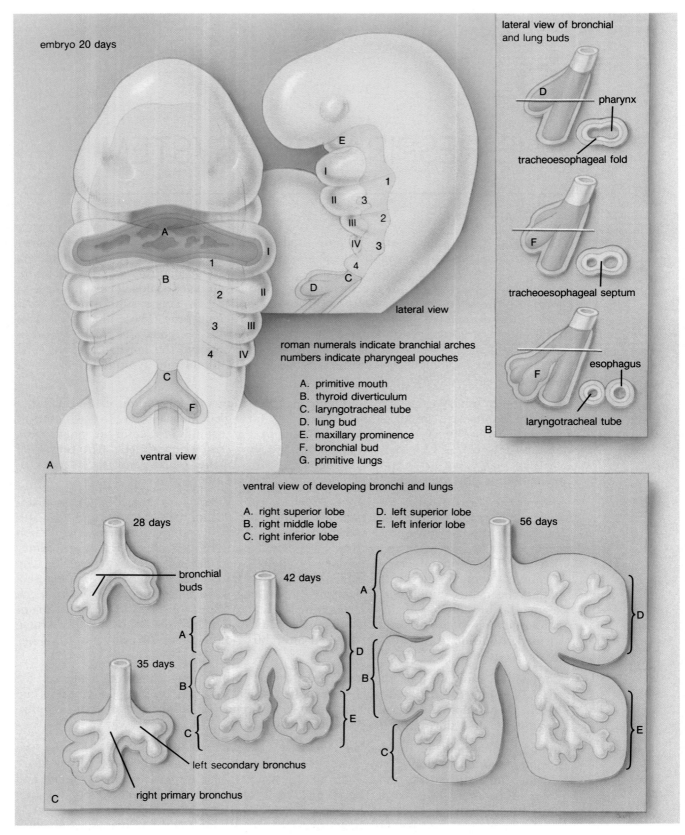

embryo 20 days

lateral view of bronchial and lung buds

D — pharynx

tracheoesophageal fold

F

tracheoesophageal septum

F — esophagus

laryngotracheal tube

E

I

II   3

III

IV   4

C

D

lateral view

1

2

3

4

A

1

B

2   II

3   III

4   IV

C

F

ventral view

A

B

roman numerals indicate branchial arches
numbers indicate pharyngeal pouches

A. primitive mouth
B. thyroid diverticulum
C. laryngotracheal tube
D. lung bud
E. maxillary prominence
F. bronchial bud
G. primitive lungs

ventral view of developing bronchi and lungs

A. right superior lobe   D. left superior lobe
B. right middle lobe   E. left inferior lobe
C. right inferior lobe

28 days

bronchial buds

35 days

42 days

56 days

A

B

C

D

E

A

B

C

D

E

left secondary bronchus

right primary bronchus

C

Figure 8–1. Drawings illustrating various stages in the development of the respiratory system. *A,* The relationship of the branchial (pharyngeal) apparatus to the respiratory system. The laryngotracheal tube (C) opens into the primitive pharynx and its caudal end divides into two bronchial buds (F). *B,* Early development of the lung bud into the bronchial buds and primitive lungs. Division of the laryngotracheal tube into the trachea and esophagus is also illustrated. *C,* Successive stages in the development of the bronchi and lungs from the fourth to eight weeks.

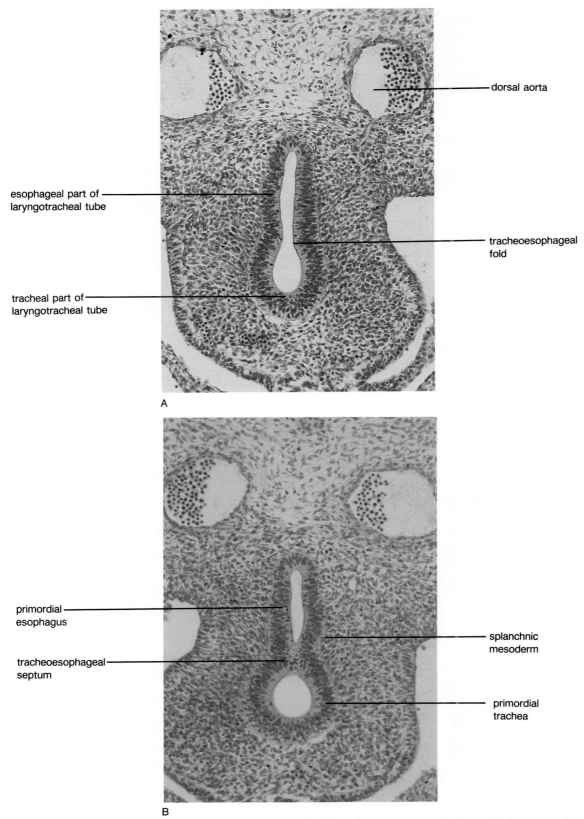

Figure 8-2. Photomicrographs of sections through an embryo (× 50) at Carnegie stage 16, about 40 days, showing division of the laryngotracheal tube into the primordia of the esophagus and trachea (see also Fig. 8–1*B*). The endoderm of the tube gives rise to the tracheal epithelium and glands and the splanchnic mesoderm gives rise to the cartilage, connective tissues and muscles of the trachea (see Fig. 8–3). *A*, Formation of the tracheoesophageal fold. *B*, Fusion of the tracheoesophageal fold to form the primordia of the trachea and esophagus.

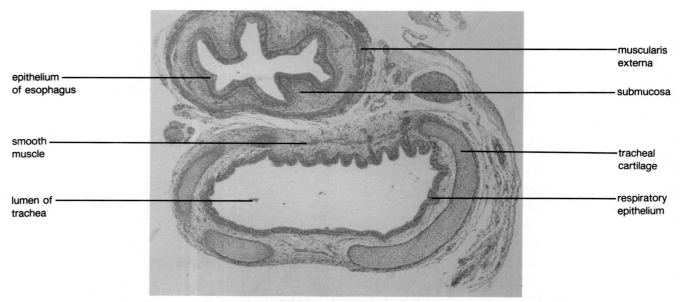

epithelium
of esophagus

smooth
muscle

lumen of
trachea

muscularis
externa

submucosa

tracheal
cartilage

respiratory
epithelium

Figure 8-3. Photomicrograph of a transverse section of the developing esophagus and trachea at 14 weeks (× 50). The respiratory epithelium is derived from the endoderm of the laryngotracheal tube and the cartilage, connective tissue and smooth muscle differentiate from the splanchnic mesoderm surrounding the laryngotracheal tube.

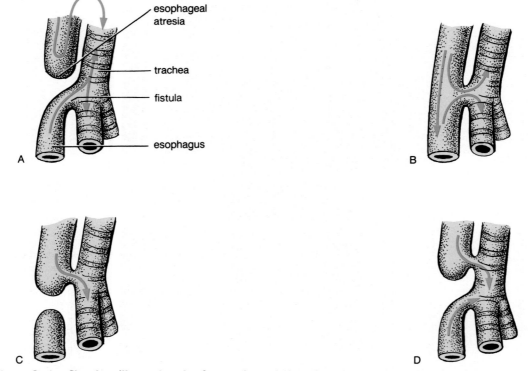

esophageal
atresia

trachea

fistula

esophagus

Figure 8-4. Sketches illustrating the four main varieties of tracheoesophageal fistula. Possible direction(s) of flow of contents is indicated by arrows. Esophageal atresia, as illustrated in *A*, is associated with tracheoesophageal fistula in about 85 per cent of cases. The abdomen rapidly becomes distended as the intestines fill with air. In *C*, air cannot enter the lower esophagus and stomach.

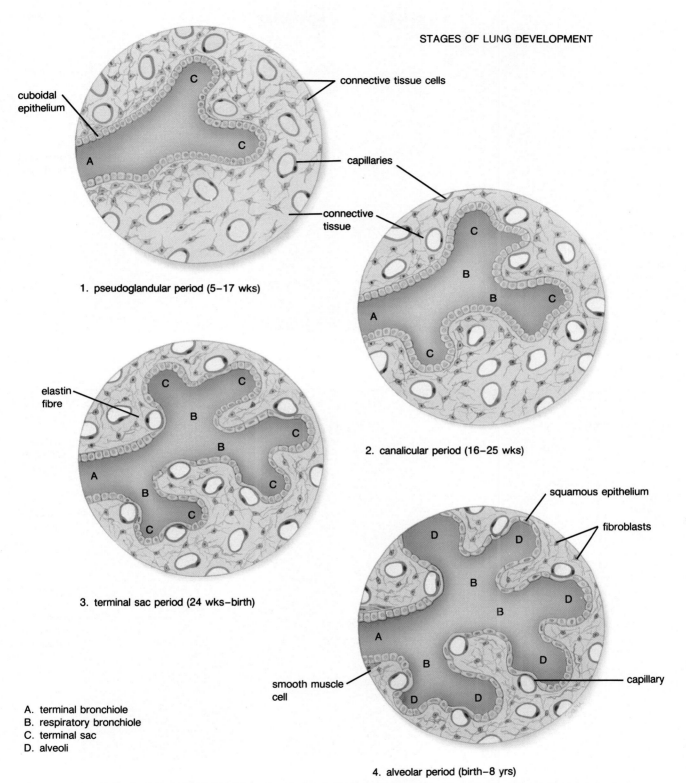

STAGES OF LUNG DEVELOPMENT

1. pseudoglandular period (5–17 wks)

2. canalicular period (16–25 wks)

3. terminal sac period (24 wks–birth)

4. alveolar period (birth–8 yrs)

cuboidal epithelium

connective tissue cells

capillaries

connective tissue

elastin fibre

squamous epithelium

fibroblasts

smooth muscle cell

capillary

A. terminal bronchiole
B. respiratory bronchiole
C. terminal sac
D. alveoli

Figure 8–5. Diagrammatic sketches of histologic sections illustrating progressive stages of lung development. 1, Pseudoglandular period (about eight weeks). 2, Late canalicular period (about 24 weeks). 3, Early terminal sac period (about 26 weeks). 4, Newborn infant. Early alveolar period. Note that the alveolocapillary membrane is thin and that some of the capillaries have begun to bulge into the primordial alveoli.

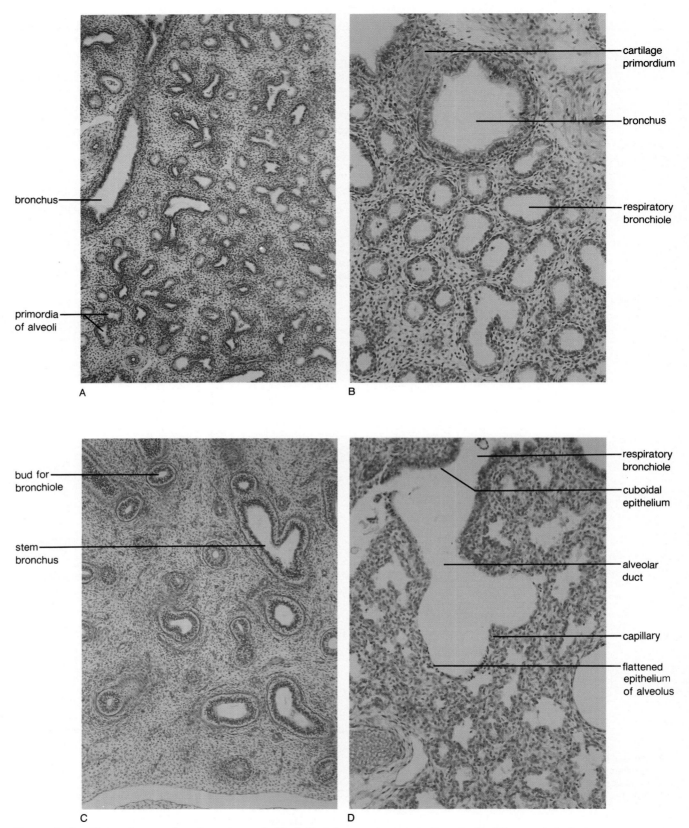

Figure 8–6. Photomicrographs of sections of developing human lungs. *A*, Pseudoglandular period, 8 weeks. Note the "glandular" appearance of the lung at this stage. *B*, Canalicular period, 16 weeks. The lumina of the bronchi and terminal bronchioles are enlarging. *C*, Canalicular period, 18 weeks. Note that many blood vessels are developing in the mesenchyme surrounding the sections of bronchi and terminal bronchioles. *D*, Terminal sac period, 24 weeks. Observe the thin-walled terminal sacs (primitive alveoli) that have developed at the ends of the respiratory bronchioles. Also observe that the number of blood vessels has increased and that some of them are closely associated with the terminal sacs or primordial alveoli.

The *alveolar period,* the final stage of lung development, occurs from the late fetal period to about eight years of age. The number of respiratory bronchioles and primitive alveoli increases.

The respiratory system develops so that it is capable of immediate function at birth. To be capable of respiration, the lungs must acquire an *alveolocapillary membrane* that is sufficiently thin, and an adequate amount of *surfactant* must be present. Pulmonary surfactant is secreted by type II alveolar cells which develop by 20 weeks. A deficiency of surfactant appears to be responsible for the failure of primitive alveoli to remain open, resulting in *hyaline membrane disease* (HMD), a major cause of the *respiratory distress syndrome* (RDS). Growth of the lungs after birth results mainly from an increase in the number of respiratory bronchioles and alveoli. New alveoli form for at least eight years after birth.

9
THE DIGESTIVE SYSTEM

The primitive or **primordial gut** (foregut, midgut, and hindgut) forms during the fourth week from the part of the *yolk sac* that is incorporated into the embryo (see Fig. 6–2). The endoderm of the primordial gut gives rise to the epithelial lining of most of the digestive tract and biliary passages, together with the parenchyma of its glands including the liver and pancreas. The epithelium at the cranial and caudal extremities of the digestive tract is derived from the ectoderm of the stomodeum and proctodeum, respectively. The muscular and connective tissue components of the digestive tract are derived from the splanchnic mesenchyme surrounding the primordial gut.

The **foregut** gives rise to the pharynx, lower respiratory system, esophagus, stomach, duodenum (proximal to the opening of the bile duct), liver, pancreas, and biliary apparatus (Figs. 9–1 to 9–3). Because the trachea and esophagus have a common origin from the foregut, incomplete partitioning by the tracheoesophageal septum results in stenoses or atresias, with or without fistulas between them (see Fig. 8–4). *Congenital duodenal atresia* results from failure of the vacuolization and recanalization process to occur following the normal solid stage of the duodenal development. Usually these epithelial cells degenerate and the lumen of the duodenum is restored.

The *hepatic diverticulum* is an outgrowth of the endodermal epithelial lining of the foregut. The epithelial liver cords and primordia of the *biliary system* develop from the hepatic diverticulum between the layers of the *ventral mesentery,* which is derived from the septum transversum (see Fig. 6–2A). These primordial cells differentiate into the *parenchyma of the liver* and the lining of the ducts of the biliary system. The fibrous and hemopoietic tissues of the liver are derived from mesenchyme in the septum transversum.

The *pancreas* is formed by dorsal and ventral *pancreatic buds* that originate from the endodermal lining of the foregut (Figs. 9–2A to C and 9–5). As the duodenum rotates to the right, the ventral pancreatic bud moves dorsally and fuses with the dorsal pancreatic bud. The *ventral pancreatic bud* forms most of the head of the pancreas, including the uncinate process. The *dorsal pancreatic bud* forms the remainder of the pancreas. In some fetuses the duct systems of the two buds fail to fuse, and an *accessory pancreatic duct* forms.

The **midgut** gives rise to the duodenum (distal to the bile duct), jejunum, ileum, cecum, vermiform appendix, ascending colon, and the right half to two thirds of the transverse colon. The midgut forms a U-shaped intestinal loop that herniates into the proximal part of the umbilical cord during the sixth week because there is no room for it in the abdomen (Figs. 9–2A and 9–3). While in the umbilical cord, the *midgut loop* rotates counterclockwise through 90 degrees. During the tenth week, the intestines rapidly return to the abdomen, rotating a further 180 degrees during this process (Fig. 9–2C).

The **hindgut** gives rise to the left one third to one half of the transverse colon, the descending and sigmoid colon, the rectum, and the superior part of the anal canal (Fig. 9–2). The inferior part of the anal canal develops from the proctodeum (anal pit). The expanded caudal part of the hindgut, known as the *cloaca,* is divided by the

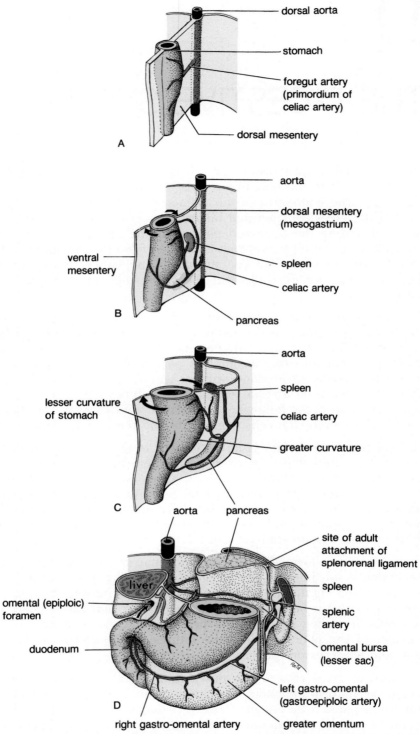

Figure 9-1. Drawings illustrating development of the stomach and duodenum and the structures associated with them (liver, spleen, and pancreas). *A,* About 24 days. The foregut artery passes between the layers of the dorsal mesentery. Observe that the stomach is fusiform at this stage. *B,* About 35 days. The spleen is developing from a mass of mesenchymal cells located between the layers of this mesentery. The pancreas develops as outgrowths from the foregut. *C,* About 40 days. Note that the dorsal mesogastrium has been carried to the left during rotation of the stomach. *D,* About 48 days. Rotation of the stomach has resulted in formation of the omental bursa (lesser sac of peritoneum). Note that the stomach and duodenum are attached to the liver by the ventral mesentery. The liver develops from an outgrowth from the caudal part of the foregut. (From Moore KL and Persaud TVN: *The Developing Human,* ed 5. Philadelphia, WB Saunders, 1993.)

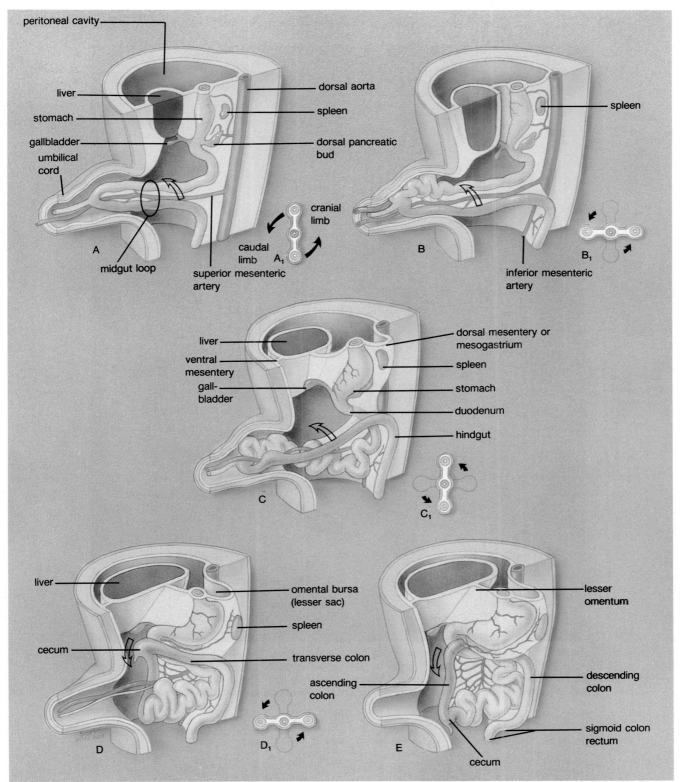

Figure 9–2. Schematic drawings illustrating rotation of the midgut as seen from the left. *A,* Around the beginning of the sixth week, showing the midgut loop partially within the umbilical cord. Note the elongated, double-layered dorsal mesentery containing the superior mesenteric artery. *A₁,* Transverse section through the midgut loop illustrating the initial relationship of the limbs of the midgut loop to the artery. *B,* Later stage showing the beginning of midgut rotation *(arrows).* Note that the cranial limb of the midgut has developed into intestines. *B₁,* Illustrates the 90-degree counterclockwise rotation that carries the cranial limb of the midgut to the right. *C,* About 10 weeks, showing the intestines returning to the abdomen. *C₁,* Illustrates a further rotation of 90 degrees. *D,* About 11 weeks, after return of intestines to the abdomen. *D₁,* Shows a further 90-degree rotation of the gut, for a total of 270 degrees. *E,* Late fetal period, showing the cecum rotating to its normal position in the lower right quadrant of the abdomen.

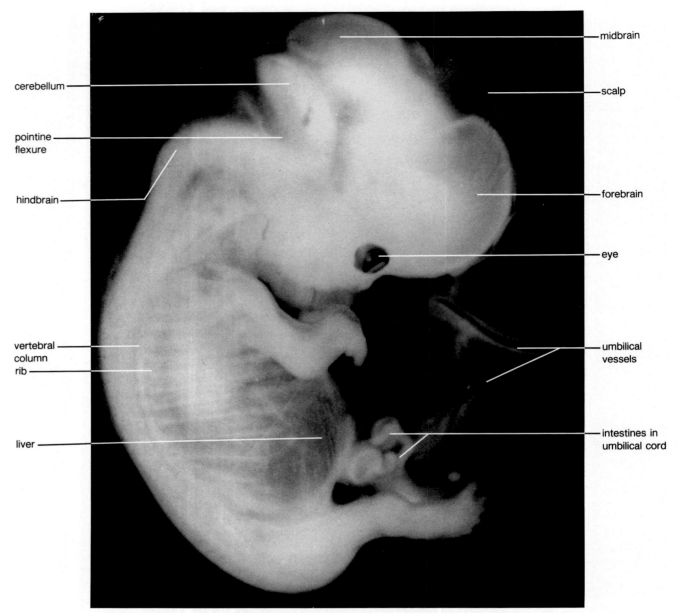

cerebellum

pointine
flexure

hindbrain

vertebral
column
rib

liver

midbrain

scalp

forebrain

eye

umbilical
vessels

intestines in
umbilical cord

Figure 9-3.   Photograph of a human embryo at Carnegie stage 23, about 56 days. Note the herniated intestine derived from the midgut loop in the proximal part of the umbilical cord. Also note the umbilical blood vessels. Because the abdomen and pelvis are poorly developed at this stage (eight weeks) the intestines herniate into the umbilical cord. They return during the tenth week (Fig. 9-2C).

urorectal septum into the urogenital sinus and rectum (Fig. 9-8). The urogenital sinus gives rise to the urinary bladder and urethra (see Chapter 10). At first, the rectum and the superior part of the anal canal are separated from the exterior by the *anal membrane,* but this membrane normally breaks down by the end of the eighth week.

Omphaloceles (Fig. 9-12), malrotations, and abnormalities of fixation of the intestine result from failure of return or abnormal rotation of the intestine in the abdomen. The intestines return from the umbilical cord by the tenth week.

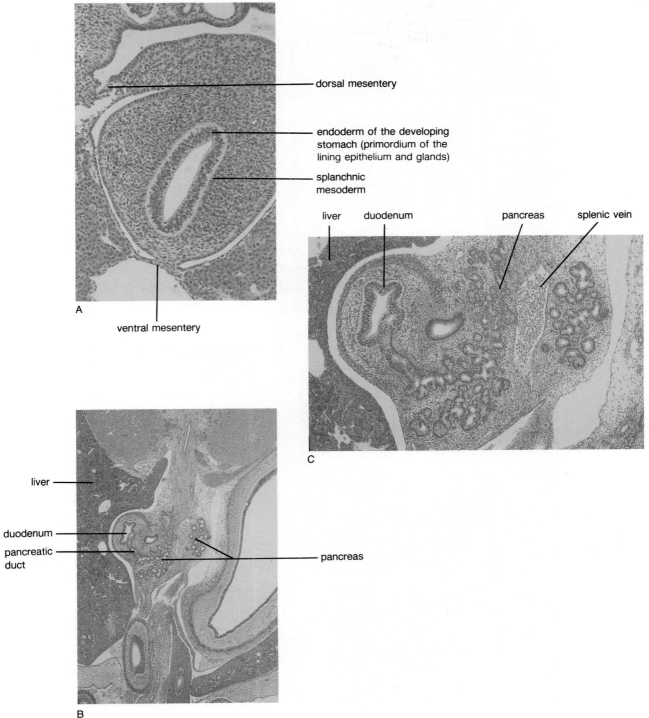

Figure 9-4. Photomicrographs of sections of the developing stomach, duodenum, and pancreas in an embryo at Carnegie stage 21, about 52 days. *A,* The stomach and its mesenteries (×160). *B,* The duodenum and pancreas (×20). *C,* Higher power view of the structures shown in *B* (×50).

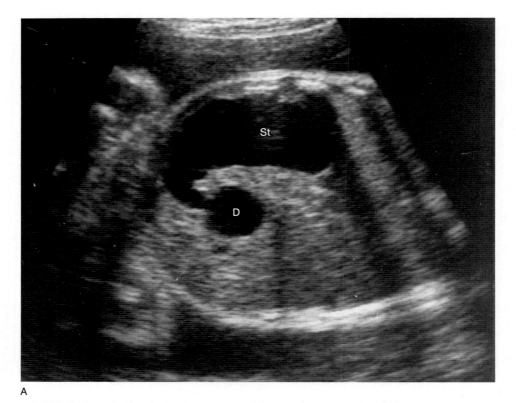

A

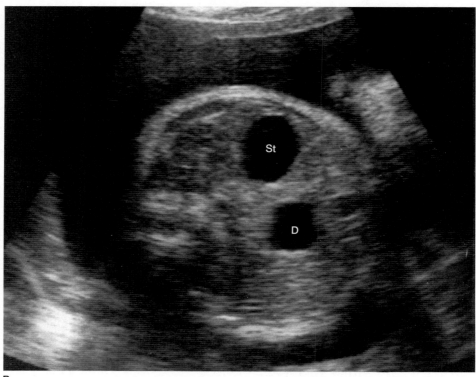

B

Figure 9–5. Ultrasound scans of a fetus at 33 weeks of gestation (31 weeks after fertilization) showing duodenal atresia. *A,* An oblique section showing the dilated, fluid-filled stomach (St) entering the proximal duodenum (D), which is also enlarged due to the atresia (blockage) distal to it. *B,* Transverse section illustrating the characteristic ''double bubble'' appearance of the stomach and duodenum when there is duodenal atresia. Duodenal atresia occurs in 1 in 10,000 live births. This anomaly is due to failure of recanalization of the duodenum which normally occurs at 10 weeks of gestation (8 weeks after fertilization). Duodenal atresia is associated with other anomalies in 48 per cent of cases: 30 per cent in infants with Down syndrome; 22 per cent in cases of gut malrotation; 20 per cent in infants with congenital heart defects. Duodenal atresia is associated with polyhydramnios in 45 per cent of cases due to the failure of absorption of swallowed amniotic fluid. (Courtesy of Dr. Lyndon M. Hill, Magee-Women's Hospital, Pittsburgh, Pennsylvania).

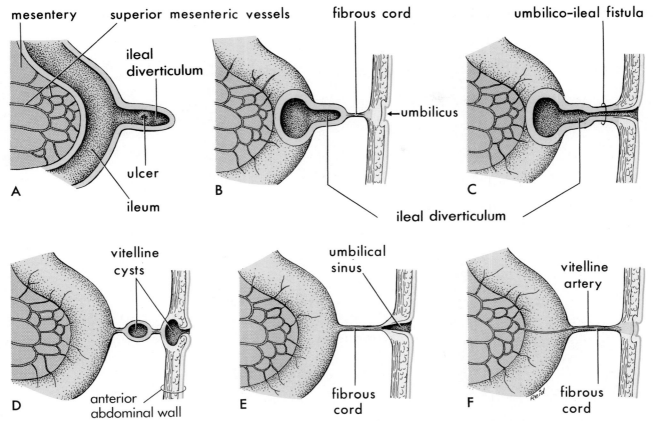

Figure 9-6. Drawings illustrating an ileal (Meckel's) diverticulum and other remnants of the yolk stalk. *A*, Section of the ileum and a diverticulum with an ulcer. *B*, Diverticulum connected to the umbilicus by a fibrous cord. *C*, Umbilico-ileal fistula resulting from persistence of the entire intra-abdominal portion of the yolk stalk. *D*, Vitelline cysts at the umbilicus and in a fibrous remnant of the yolk stalk. *E*, Umbilical sinus resulting from the persistence of the yolk stalk near the umbilicus. *F*, The yolk stalk has persisted as a fibrous cord connecting the ileum with the umbilicus. A persistent vitelline artery extends along the fibrous cord to the umbilicus. (From Moore KL and Persaud TVN: *The Developing Human,* ed 5. Philadelphia, WB Saunders, 1993.)

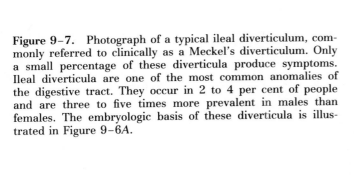

Figure 9-7. Photograph of a typical ileal diverticulum, commonly referred to clinically as a Meckel's diverticulum. Only a small percentage of these diverticula produce symptoms. Ileal diverticula are one of the most common anomalies of the digestive tract. They occur in 2 to 4 per cent of people and are three to five times more prevalent in males than females. The embryologic basis of these diverticula is illustrated in Figure 9-6A.

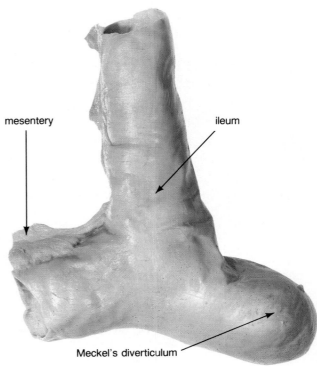

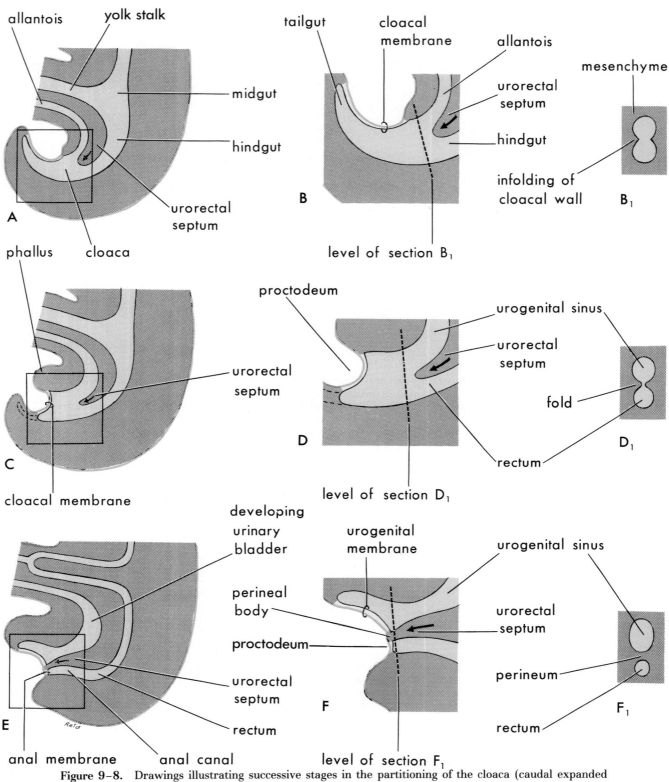

Figure 9–8. Drawings illustrating successive stages in the partitioning of the cloaca (caudal expanded part of hindgut) into the rectum and urogenital sinus by the urorectal septum. *A*, *C*, and *E*, are views from the left side at four, six, and seven weeks, respectively. *B*, *D*, and *F* are enlargements of the cloacal region. *B₁*, *D₁*, and *F₁* are transverse sections through the cloaca at the levels shown in *B*, *D*, and *F*. (From Moore KL and Persaud TVN: *The Developing Human*, ed 5. Philadelphia, WB Saunders, 1993.)

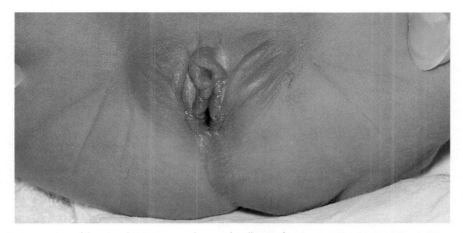

Figure 9-9. Female neonate with membranous anal atresia (imperforate anus). A tracheoesophageal fistula was also present (see Fig. 8-4). In most cases of anal atresia, a thin layer of tissue separates the anal canal from the exterior (Fig. 9-10C). This anomaly is due to failure of the anal membrane to perforate at the end of the eighth week. Some form of imperforate anus occurs about once in every 5000 neonates; it is more common in males. (Courtesy of Dr. A.E. Chudley, Children's Centre, Winnipeg, Manitoba, Canada.)

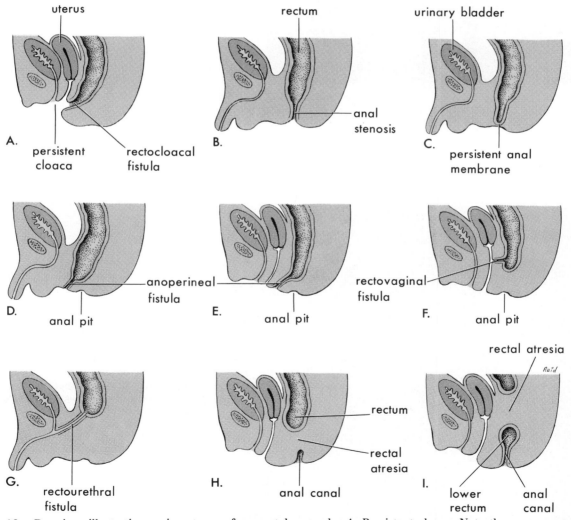

Figure 9-10. Drawings illustrating various types of anorectal anomaly. *A,* Persistent cloaca. Note the common outlet for the intestinal, urinary, and reproductive tracts. *B,* Anal stenosis. *C,* Membranous anal atresia (covered anus). *D* and *E,* Anal agenesis with a perineal fistula. *F,* Anorectal agenesis with a rectovaginal fistula. *G,* Anorectal agenesis with a rectourethral fistula. *H* and *I,* Rectal atresia. (From Moore KL and Persaud TVN: *The Developing Human,* ed 5. Philadelphia, WB Saunders, 1993.)

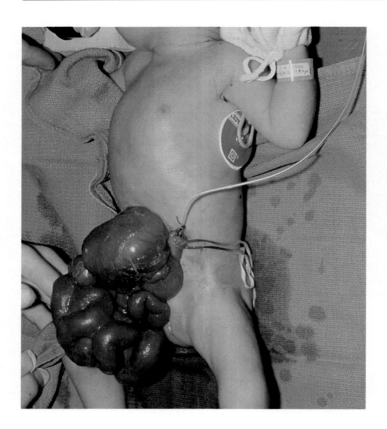

Figure 9–11. Neonate with an anterior abdominal wall defect known as gastroschisis. The defect was relatively small (2 to 4 cm) and involved all layers of the abdominal wall. It was located to the right of the umbilicus. The generally accepted etiology of gastroschisis is that the defect is due to abnormal involution of the right umbilical vein which occurs during the fifth week. Most infants with this severe anomaly now survive due to improved perinatal management. Gastroschisis should not be confused with omphalocele (Fig. 9–12). (Courtesy of Dr. A.E. Chudley, Children's Centre, Winnipeg, Manitoba, Canada.)

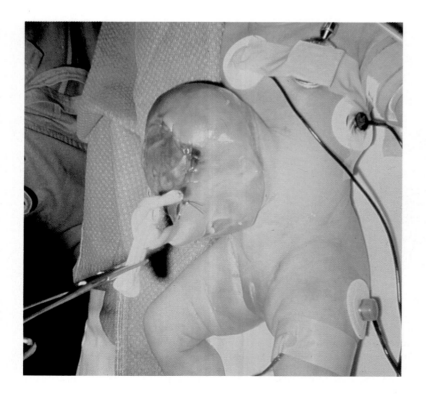

Figure 9–12. Neonate with a giant-type omphalocele due to a median defect of the abdominal muscles, fascia, and skin at the umbilicus that resulted in the herniation of intra-abdominal structures (liver and intestine) into the proximal end of the umbilical cord. It is covered by a membrane composed of peritoneum and amnion. In some cases, omphalocele may be a persistence of the normal embryonic stage of umbilical herniation (Fig. 9–3). (Courtesy of Dr. N.E. Wiseman, Pediatric Surgeon, Children's Centre, Winnipeg, Manitoba, Canada).

Because the gut is normally occluded during the fifth and sixth weeks due to rapid mitotic activity of its epithelium, *stenosis* (partial obstruction), *atresia* (complete obstruction), and duplications result if recanalization fails to occur or occurs abnormally (Fig. 9–5). Various remnants of the yolk stalk may persist. *Ileal (Meckel's) diverticula* are common, but only a few of them become inflamed and produce pain (Fig. 9–6). Most ileal diverticula develop from remnants of the yolk stalk (Fig. 9–7).

Anorectal anomalies usually result from abnormal partitioning of the cloaca by the urorectal septum into the rectum and anal canal posteriorly and the urinary bladder and urethra anteriorly (Fig. 9–8). Arrested growth and/or deviation of the urorectal septum in a dorsal direction causes most of the anorectal abnormalities, such as rectal atresia and abnormal connections (fistulas) between the rectum and the urethra, urinary bladder, or vagina.

10

THE UROGENITAL SYSTEM

The urogenital system develops from three sources: (1) intermediate mesoderm, (2) mesothelium (coelomic epithelium) lining the peritoneal cavity, and (3) endoderm of the urogenital sinus (Fig. 10–1). Three successive sets of **kidneys** develop: (1) the nonfunctional *pronephroi,* (2) the *mesonephroi,* which serve as temporary excretory organs, and (3) the functional *metanephroi* or permanent kidneys (Fig. 10–2).

The metanephroi develop from two sources: (1) the *metanephric diverticulum or ureteric bud,* which gives rise to the ureter, renal pelvis, calices, and collecting tubules, and (2) the *metanephric mesoderm,* which gives rise to the nephrons (Figs. 10–2 to 10–4). At first the **kidneys** are located in the pelvis but they gradually "ascend" to the abdomen. This apparent migration results from disproportionate growth of the lumbar and sacral regions.

The **urinary bladder** develops from the urogenital sinus and the surrounding splanchnic mesenchyme (see Figure 9–8). The female urethra and almost all of the male urethra have a similar origin. The cortex and medulla of the suprarenal or adrenal glands have different origins (Figs. 10–5 to 10–7 and 10–11). The cortex develops from mesoderm and the medulla develops from neural crest cells.

Developmental abnormalities of the kidneys and ureters are common (Fig. 10–8 to 10–10). Incomplete division of the metanephric diverticulum results in partial or complete *duplication of the ureter* (Fig. 10–10) and/or a supernumerary kidney. Failure of the kidney to "ascend" from its embryonic pelvic position results in *ectopic kidney* that is abnormally rotated, e.g., **pelvic kidney** (Fig. 10–8).

The genital or reproductive system develops in close association with the urinary or excretory system (Fig. 10–11). *Genetic sex* is established at fertilization, but the gonads do not begin to attain sexual characteristics until the seventh week (Figs. 10–12 to 10–14). The *primordial germ cells* form in the wall of the yolk sac during the fourth week and migrate into the developing gonads and differentiate into the definitive germ cells (oogonia/spermatogonia). The external genitalia do not acquire distinct masculine or feminine characteristics until the twelfth week (Fig. 10–17).

The reproductive organs develop from primordia that are identical in both sexes. During this indifferent or *undifferentiated stage* an embryo has the potential to develop into either a male or a female (Fig. 10–11). Gonadal sex is determined by the *testis-determining factor (TDF) on the Y chromosome.* TDF is located in the sex-determining region of the short arm of the Y chromosome (SRY).

TDF directs testicular differentiation. The Leydig cells produce testosterone that stimulates development of the mesonephric ducts into male genital ducts (Figs. 10–11 and 10–15). These androgens also stimulate development of the indifferent external genitalia into the penis and scrotum (Fig. 10–17). A *müllerian inhibiting factor* (MIF), produced by the Sertoli cells of the testes, inhibits development of the paramesonephric ducts (Fig. 10–15).

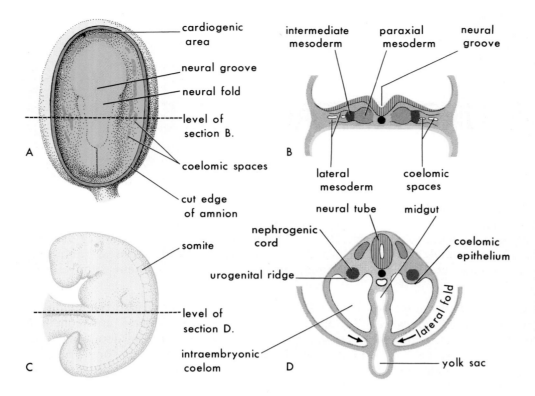

Figure 10–1. *A,* Dorsal view of an embryo during the third week (Carnegie stage 9, about 19 days). *B,* Transverse section through the embryo showing the position of the intermediate mesoderm before lateral folding of the embryo. *C,* Lateral view of an embryo during the fourth week (about 26 days). *D,* Transverse section through the embryo showing the urogenital ridges produced by the nephrogenic cords of mesoderm derived from the intermediate mesoderm. (From Moore KL and Persaud TVN: *The Developing Human,* ed 5. Philadelphia, WB Saunders, 1993.)

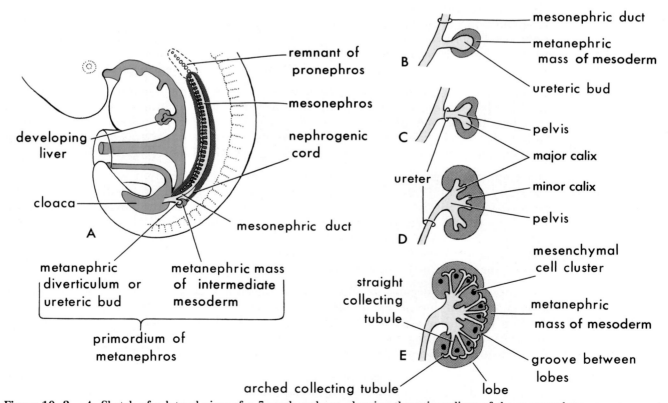

Figure 10–2. *A,* Sketch of a lateral view of a 5-week embryo, showing the primordium of the metanephros or permanent kidney. Note that the pronephric kidney has degenerated and that its duct has become the duct of the mesonephric kidney. *B* to *E,* Sketches showing successive stages in the development of the metanephric diverticulum or ureteric bud (fifth to eighth weeks). Observe the development of the ureter, renal pelvis, calices, and collecting tubules. The renal lobes, illustrated in *E,* are visible in the kidneys of the 9-week fetus (Fig. 10–7). (From Moore KL and Persaud TVN: *The Developing Human,* ed 5. Philadelphia, WB Saunders, 1993.)

Figure 10-3. Diagrammatic sketches illustrating progressive stages in the development of nephrons. Note that the metanephric tubules, the primordia of the nephrons, become continuous with the collecting tubules to form uriniferous tubules. This process commences around the beginning of the eighth week. It has been estimated that by 11 to 13 weeks, approximately 20 per cent of nephrons are relatively mature. This is when urine formation begins. The number of nephrons more than doubles from 20 weeks to 38 weeks of gestation. Urine formation continues throughout fetal life. It is excreted into the amniotic sac and forms a major component of the amniotic fluid. A mature fetus swallows several hundred milliliters of amniotic fluid daily. This fluid is absorbed by the intestines and passes in the fetal blood to the placenta for transfer to the maternal blood for elimination of water and waste products by her kidneys. (From Moore KL and Persaud TVN: *The Developing Human,* ed 5. Philadelphia, WB Saunders, 1993.)

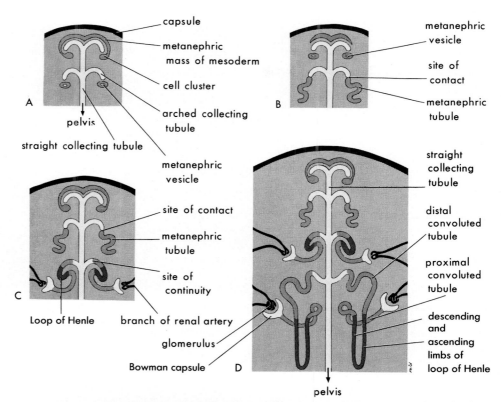

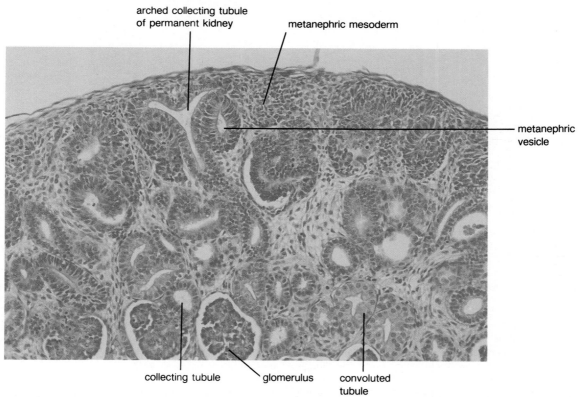

Figure 10-4. Photomicrograph of a section of the metanephric kidney of an 11-week fetus (×200). These kidneys begin to develop late in the fifth week (Fig. 10-2).

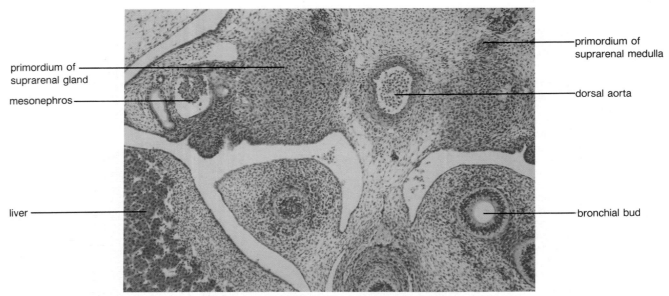

primordium of suprarenal gland

mesonephros

liver

primordium of suprarenal medulla

dorsal aorta

bronchial bud

Figure 10-5. Photomicrograph of a section of an embryo at Carnegie stage 17, about 42 days, primarily to show the developing suprarenal (adrenal) glands. Observe that the developing cortex of each gland is large, whereas the small medulla lies dorsal to the cortex (see also Figure 10-11). The medullary cells, derived from neural crest cells, are later engulfed by the cortex and are located inside the cortex.

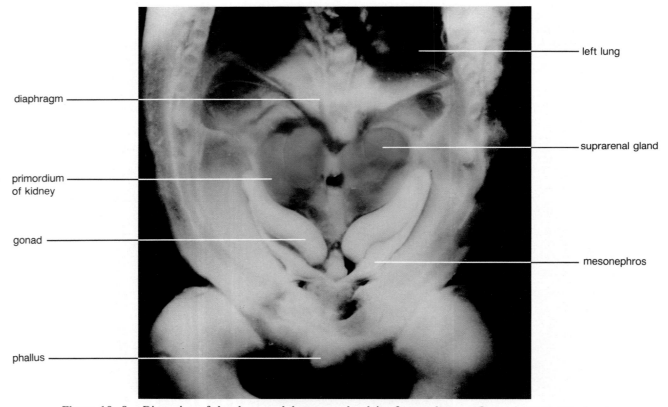

diaphragm

primordium of kidney

gonad

phallus

left lung

suprarenal gland

mesonephros

Figure 10-6. Dissection of the thorax, abdomen, and pelvis of an embryo at Carnegie stage 22, about 54 days. (For the external appearance and size of an embryo at this stage, see Fig. 2-24). Observe the large suprarenal (adrenal) glands and the elongated mesonephros (mesonephric kidney). Also observe the gonads (testes or ovaries). The sex of these glands is not obvious in an external view such as this (see Fig. 10-14). External evidence of sex is not recognizable either. The phallus will develop into a penis or a clitoris depending on the genetic sex of the embryo. (From Nishimura H (ed): *Atlas of Human Prenatal Histology.* Tokyo, Igaku-Shoin, 1983).

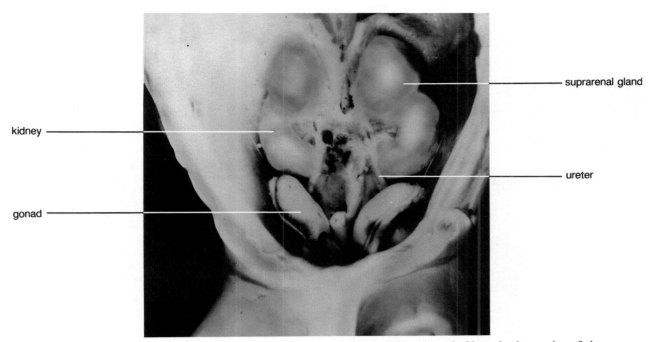

kidney ——————

gonad ——————

—— suprarenal gland

—— ureter

Figure 10-7. Dissection of the abdomen of a 9-week fetus, (CRL 41 mm). Note the large size of the suprarenal or adrenal glands. These glands normally reduce to their normal size during the first two weeks after birth.

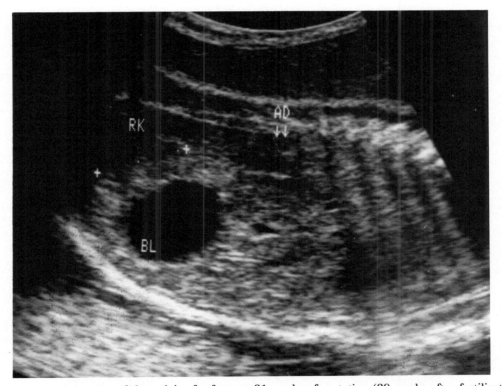

Figure 10-8. Sonogram of the pelvis of a fetus at 31 weeks of gestation (29 weeks after fertilization). Observe the abnormally low position of the right kidney (RK) near the urinary bladder (BL). This abnormal pelvic kidney resulted from its failure to "ascend" during the sixth to ninth weeks. Also observe the suprarenal or adrenal gland (AD), which develops separately from the kidney. When the kidneys "ascend" into the abdomen, these glands lie at their superior poles (Fig. 10-7). (Courtesy of Dr. Lyndon M. Hill, Director of Ultrasound, Magee-Women's Hospital, Pittsburgh, Pennsylvania.)

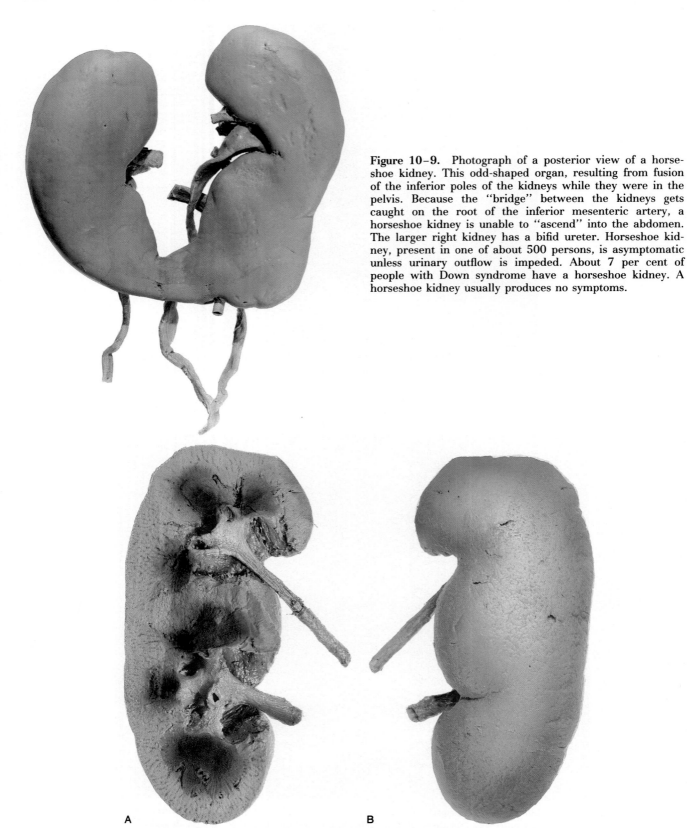

Figure 10-9. Photograph of a posterior view of a horse-shoe kidney. This odd-shaped organ, resulting from fusion of the inferior poles of the kidneys while they were in the pelvis. Because the "bridge" between the kidneys gets caught on the root of the inferior mesenteric artery, a horseshoe kidney is unable to "ascend" into the abdomen. The larger right kidney has a bifid ureter. Horseshoe kidney, present in one of about 500 persons, is asymptomatic unless urinary outflow is impeded. About 7 per cent of people with Down syndrome have a horseshoe kidney. A horseshoe kidney usually produces no symptoms.

A   B

Figure 10-10. Photographs of a kidney with two ureters and renal pelves. This congenital anomaly results from incomplete division of the metanephric diverticulum or ureteric bud (Fig. 10-2). *A*, Longitudinal section through the kidney showing two renal pelves. *B*, Anterior surface. Both ureters opened into the urinary bladder.

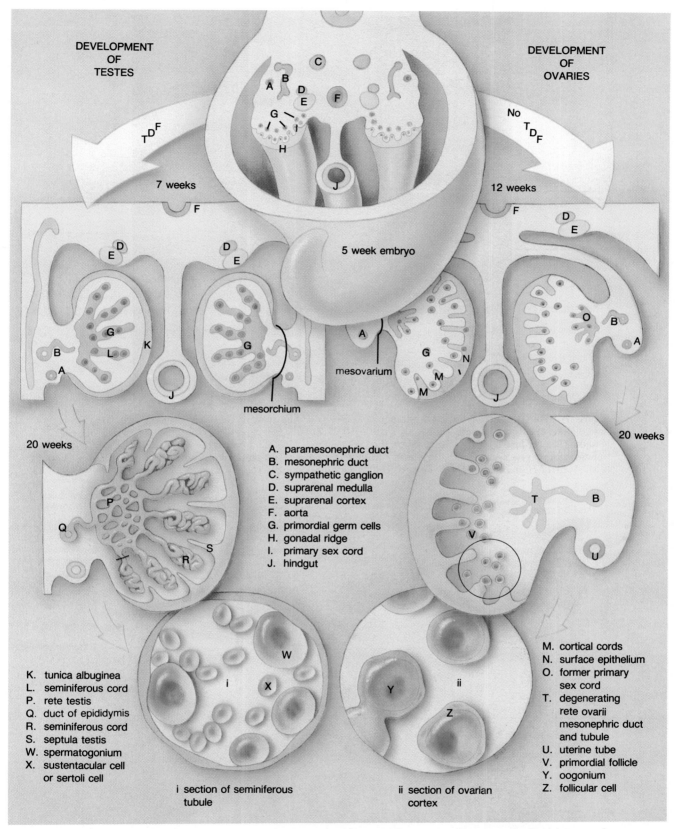

DEVELOPMENT OF TESTES

DEVELOPMENT OF OVARIES

7 weeks

12 weeks

5 week embryo

20 weeks

20 weeks

A. paramesonephric duct
B. mesonephric duct
C. sympathetic ganglion
D. suprarenal medulla
E. suprarenal cortex
F. aorta
G. primordial germ cells
H. gonadal ridge
I. primary sex cord
J. hindgut

mesovarium

mesorchium

K. tunica albuginea
L. seminiferous cord
P. rete testis
Q. duct of epididymis
R. seminiferous cord
S. septula testis
W. spermatogonium
X. sustentacular cell or sertoli cell

M. cortical cords
N. surface epithelium
O. former primary sex cord
T. degenerating rete ovarii mesonephric duct and tubule
U. uterine tube
V. primordial follicle
Y. oogonium
Z. follicular cell

i section of seminiferous tubule

ii section of ovarian cortex

Figure 10–11. Schematic illustration showing differentiation of the indifferent or sexless gonads *(top)* into ovaries or testes. *Left side* shows the development of testes resulting from the effects of the testis-determining factor (TDF) located on the Y chromosome. Note that the primary sex cords (I) become seminiferous cords (R), the primordia of the seminiferous tubules. The parts of the primary sex cords that enter the medulla of the testis form the rete testis (P). In the section of the testis at the *bottom left,* observe that there are two kinds of cells, spermatogonia (W), derived from the primordial germ cells (G) and sustentacular or Sertoli cells (X). *Right side* shows the development of ovaries in the absence of TDF. Cortical cords (M) have extended from the surface epithelium of the gonad and primordial germ cells (G) have entered them. They are the primordia of the oogonia (Y). Follicular cells (Z) are derived from the mesenchyme (primitive connective tissue) separating the oogonia (Y).

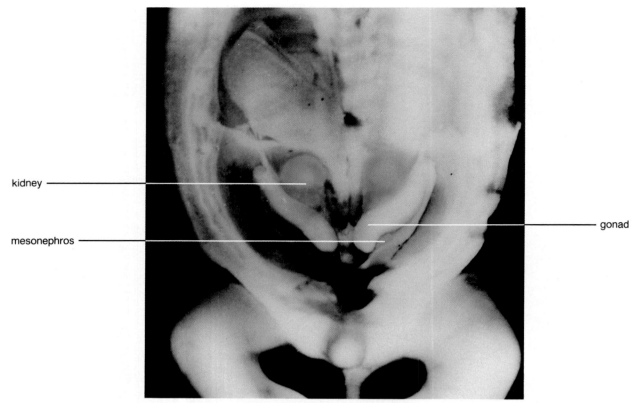

kidney

mesonephros

gonad

Figure 10-12. Dissection of the abdomen and pelvis of an embryo at Carnegie stage 22, about 54 days. The suprarenal glands shown in Figure 10-6 have been removed. Note the large size of the gonads (future testes or ovaries). Note the presence of the temporary mesonephric kidneys. They function for a few weeks and degenerate around the end of the final trimester. (From Nishimura H (ed): *Atlas of Human Prenatal Histology.* Tokyo, Igaku-Shoin, 1983).

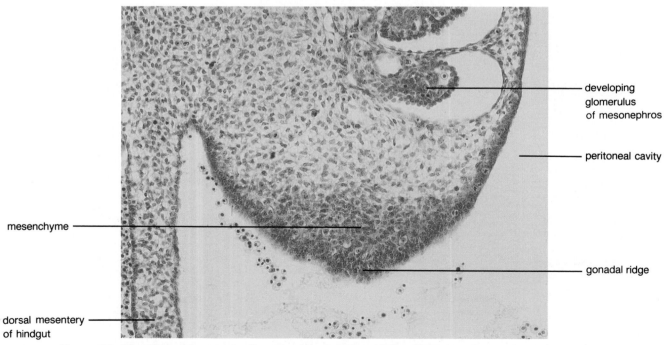

developing
glomerulus
of mesonephros

peritoneal cavity

mesenchyme

gonadal ridge

dorsal mesentery
of hindgut

Figure 10-13. Photomicrograph of a transverse section of the abdomen of an embryo at Carnegie stage 16, about 40 days, showing the gonadal (genital) ridge which will develop into a testis or an ovary depending on the genetic sex of the embryo. The sex of the embryo is not evident morphologically at this stage. (For the external appearance and size of an embryo at this stage, see Fig. 2-18). Most of the developing gonad is composed of mesenchyme derived from the coelomic epithelium of the gonadal ridge.

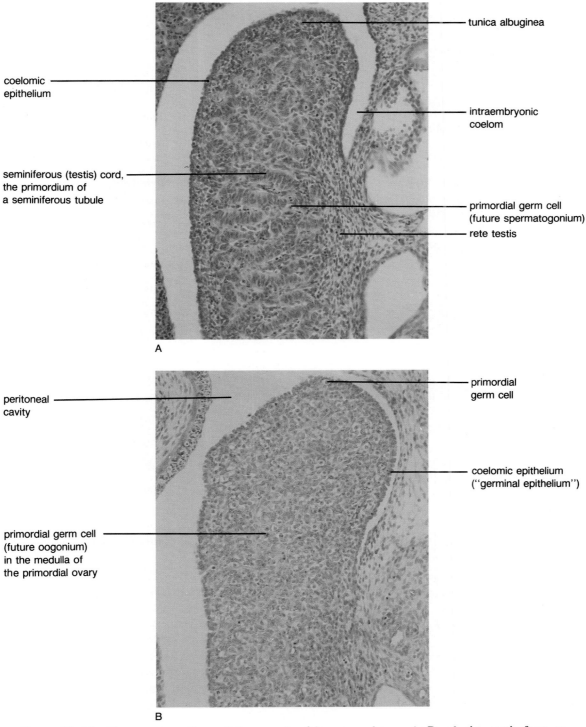

coelomic
epithelium

seminiferous (testis) cord,
the primordium of
a seminiferous tubule

tunica albuginea

intraembryonic
coelom

primordial germ cell
(future spermatogonium)

rete testis

A

peritoneal
cavity

primordial germ cell
(future oogonium)
in the medulla of
the primordial ovary

primordial
germ cell

coelomic epithelium
(''germinal epithelium'')

B

Figure 10–14. Transverse sections of the gonads of human embryos. *A*, Developing testis from an embryo at Carnegie stage 20, about 51 days. Observe the prominent seminiferous cords, the primordia of the seminiferous tubules. The large cells within them with dark nuclei are primordial germ cells, primordia of spermatogonia (see also Fig. 10–11). *B*, Developing ovary from an embryo at the same stage. The absence of seminiferous cords is a diagnostic characteristic of ovaries. The large cells with dark nuclei are primordial germ cells, the primordia of oogonia.

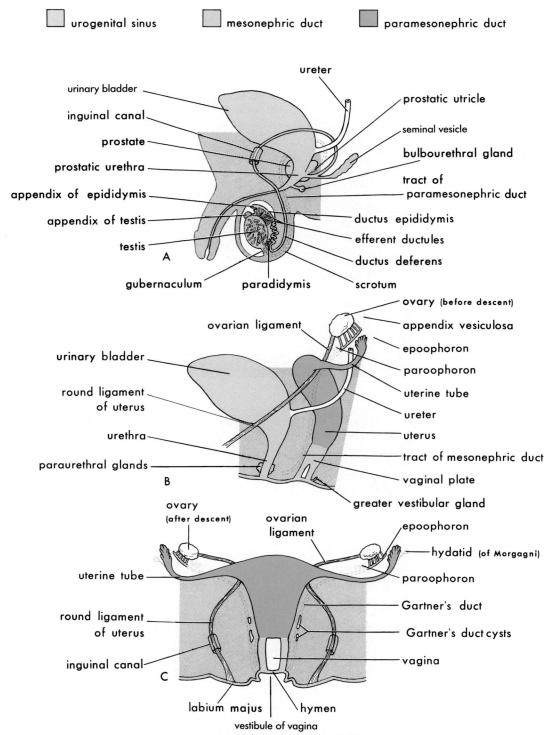

Figure 10–15.   Schematic drawings illustrating development of the male and female reproductive systems from the genital ducts and the urogenital sinus. Vestigial structures are also shown. *A,* Reproductive system in a newborn male. *B,* Female reproductive system in a 12-week fetus. *C,* Reproductive system in a newborn female. Both male and female embryos have two pairs of genital ducts. The mesonephric (wolffian) ducts play an important part in the development of the male reproductive system. In male embryos, the mesonephric ducts are stimulated to develop into male ducts by testosterone produced by the testis. A müllerian inhibiting factor (MIF) is also produced by the testis, which inhibits development of the paramesonephric ducts. The lack of testosterone and MIF in female embryos results in the development of the paramesonephric (müllerian) ducts into female structures (uterine [fallopian] tubes and uterus). Remnants of these ducts (mesonephric and paramesonephric) may give rise to vestigial structures (e.g., paradidymis in males and Gartner's ducts in females). (From Moore KL and Persaud TVN: *The Developing Human,* ed 5. Philadelphia, WB Saunders, 1993.)

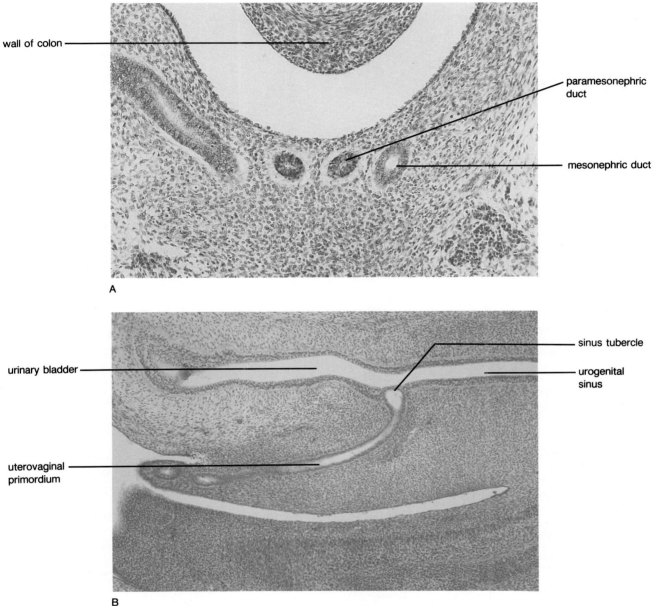

wall of colon

paramesonephric
duct

mesonephric duct

A

sinus tubercle

urinary bladder

urogenital
sinus

uterovaginal
primordium

B

Figure 10–16.   Photomicrographs of sections of human embryos. *A,* Transverse section of an embryo at Carnegie stage 22, about 54 days (×200) showing the mesonephric and paramesonephric ducts that are present in male and female embryos (see Fig. 10–15). In female fetuses, the paramesonephric ducts form the uterine (fallopian) tubes and then fuse to form the uterovaginal canal, the primordium of the uterus and vagina. *B,* Longitudinal section of a female embryo at Carnegie stage 23, about 56 days (×175), showing the uterus developing from the uterovaginal primordium formed by the fused paramesonephric (müllerian) ducts.

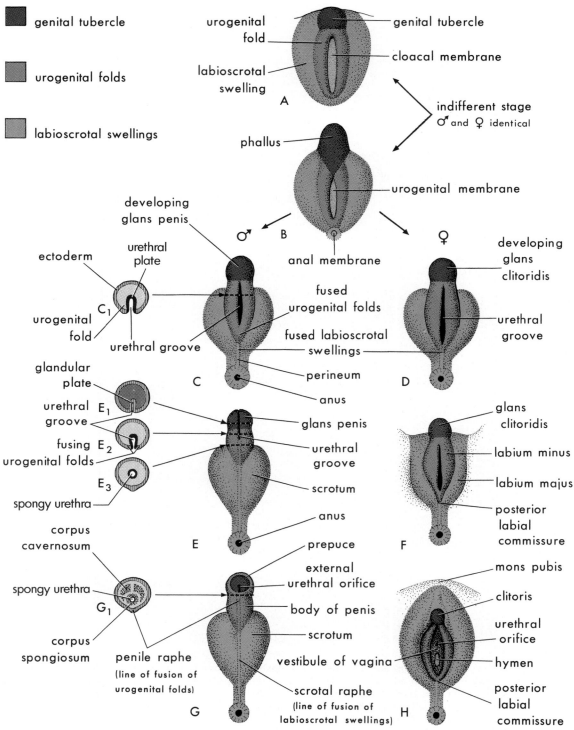

Figure 10–17. *A* and *B*, Diagrams illustrating development of the external genitalia during the indifferent stage (fourth to seventh weeks). *C, E,* and *G,* Stages in the development of male external genitalia at 9, 11, and 12 weeks, respectively. To the left are schematic transverse sections (C_1, E_1 to E_3, and G_1) through the developing penis, illustrating formation of the spongy urethra. *D, F,* and *H.* Stages in the development of female external genitalia at 9, 11, and 12 weeks, respectively. (From Moore KL and Persaud TVN: *The Developing Human,* ed 5. Philadelphia, WB Saunders, 1993.)

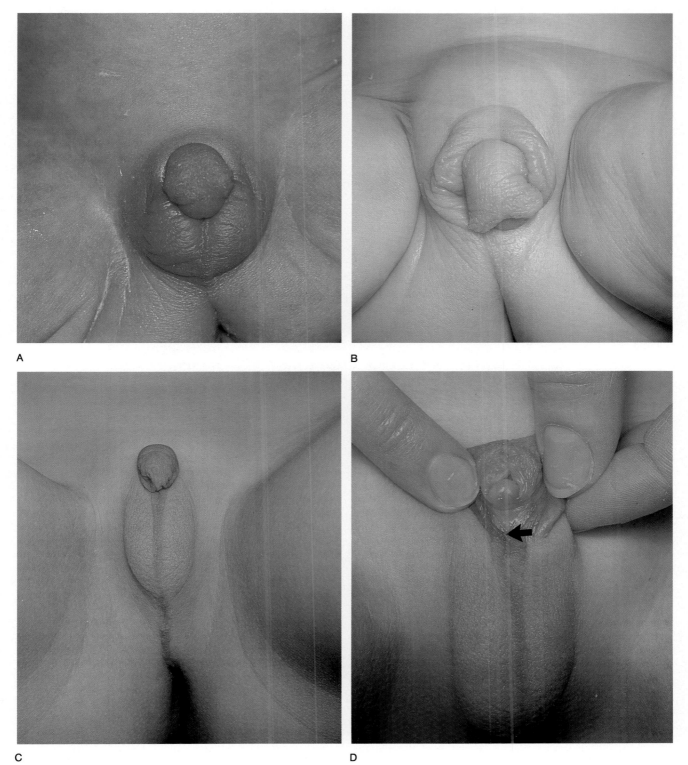

Figure 10-18. Photographs of the external genitalia of female pseudohermaphrodites resulting from congenital adrenal hyperplasia (CAH). The degree of labioscrotal fusion and clitoral hypertrophy depends upon the stage of differentiation at which the fetus is exposed to the masculinizing hormones, as well as upon the biologic potency of the androgens produced by the hyperplastic suprarenal or adrenal glands. *A,* External genitalia of a newborn female, exhibiting enlargement of the clitoris and fusion of the labia majora. *B,* External genitalia of a female infant showing considerable enlargement of the clitoris. The unfused labia majora are rugose as in a scrotum. *C* and *D,* External genitalia of a 6-year-old girl, showing an enlarged clitoris and fused labia majora that have formed a scrotum-like structure. In *D,* the clitoris has been elevated to show the location of the opening of the urogenital sinus *(arrow),* the primordium of the vestibule of the vagina.

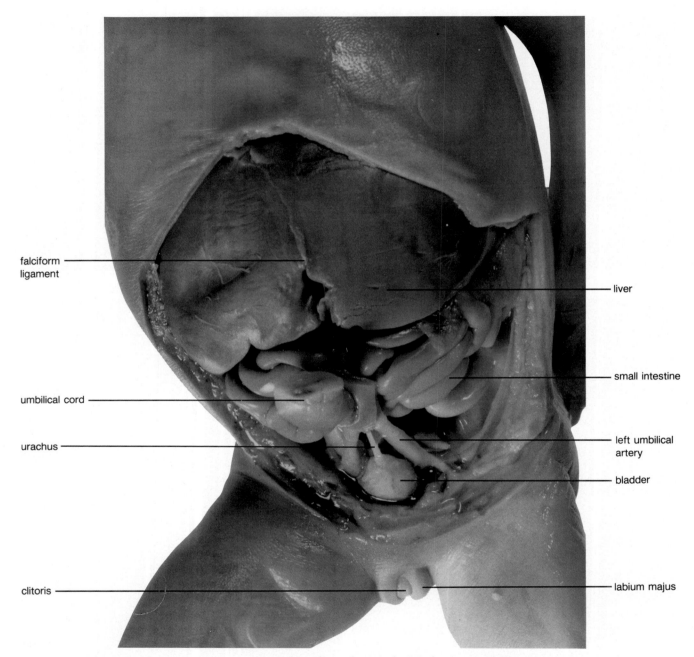

labium majus

small intestine

liver

left umbilical
artery

bladder

labium majus

falciform
ligament

umbilical cord

urachus

clitoris

Figure 10–19.   Photograph of a dissection of an 18-week female fetus, primarily to show the relationship of the urachus, a derivative of the allantois, to the urinary bladder and umbilical arteries. The urachus becomes the median umbilical ligament in adults. The umbilical arteries carry poorly oxygenated blood to the placenta. They are represented in adults by the medial umbilical ligaments. Observe that the clitoris is still relatively large at this stage. It becomes smaller as full term is approached.

In the absence of a Y chromosome (i.e., TDF and MIF) and the presence of two X chromosomes, **ovaries** develop (Fig. 10–11), the mesonephric ducts regress (Fig. 10–15), the paramesonephric ducts develop into the uterus and uterine tubes (Figs. 10–15 and 10–16), the vagina develops from the vaginal plate derived from the urogenital sinus, and the indifferent external genitalia develop into the clitoris and labia (majora and minora [Figs. 10–17 and 10–19]).

Most abnormalities of the female genital tract result from incomplete fusion of the paramesonephric ducts (e.g., double uterus). *Cryptorchidism* and ectopic testes result from abnormalities of testicular descent. In males, failure of the urogenital folds to fuse normally results in various types of *hypospadias*.

Persons with *true hermaphroditism,* an extremely rare intersexual condition, have both ovarian and testicular tissue and variable internal and external genitalia. Errors in sexual differentiation cause pseudohermaphroditism. *Male pseudohermaphroditism* results from failure of the fetal testes to produce adequate amounts of masculinizing hormones or from the tissue insensitivity of the sexual structures. *Female pseudohermaphroditism* usually results from congenital adrenal hyperplasia (CAH), a disorder of the fetal suprarenal (adrenal) glands that causes excessive production of androgens and masculinization of the external genitalia (Fig. 10–18).

Masculinization of some male fetuses fails to occur due to a resistance to the action of testosterone at the cellular level in the labioscrotal and urogenital folds (Fig. 10–17). As a result these fetuses appear as normal female infants. The developmental defect is in the androgen receptor mechanism. Testes are present in these females but they are not functional. This condition, called the *androgen insensitivity syndrome* (Moore and Persaud, 1993), was formerly referred to as the testicular feminization syndrome. The infants develop into women whose appearance and psychosexual orientation is female; however they are sterile.

11

THE CARDIOVASCULAR SYSTEM

The cardiovascular system begins to develop toward the end of the third week, and the **primordial heart** starts to beat at 21 to 22 days. Mesenchymal cells derived from splanchnic mesoderm proliferate and form isolated cell clusters, which soon develop into two endothelial tubes that join to form the primitive vascular system (Figs. 11–1 to 11–3). Paired endothelial tubes form and fuse into a single endothelial heart tube. This primitive or primordial heart tube is soon surrounded by myoblasts (muscle-forming cells), which form the *myocardium* (Fig. 11–3).

The primordium of the heart consists of four chambers: sinus venosus, atrium, ventricle, and bulbus cordis. The *truncus arteriosus* is continuous caudally with the *bulbus cordis* and enlarges cranially to form the *aortic sac* (Fig. 11–1). As the heart grows, it bends to the right and soon acquires the general external appearance of the adult heart. The heart becomes partitioned into four chambers between the fourth and seventh weeks (Figs. 11–4 and 11–5). Three systems of paired veins drain into the primordial heart (Fig. 11–1).

FATE OF THE SINUS VENOSUS.   This venous sinus is initially a separate chamber of the heart that opens into the right atrium (Figs. 13–1 and 13–3*C*). As development of the heart proceeds, the left horn of the sinus venosus becomes the *coronary sinus* and the right horn is incorporated into the wall of the right atrium where it forms the smooth portion of the adult right atrial wall. The right half of the primitive atrium persists as the *right auricle,* an appendage of the atrium.

FORMATION OF THE LEFT ATRIUM.   Most of the adult left atrium is formed by incorporation of the *primitive pulmonary vein.* As the atrium enlarges, parts of this vein and its branches are absorbed, with the result that four pulmonary veins eventually enter the adult atrium. The smooth-walled part of the left atrium is derived from absorbed pulmonary vein tissue, whereas the left auricle (auricular appendage) is derived from the primitive atrium.

During the fourth and fifth weeks, the primordial heart is divided into a four-chambered organ (Figs. 11–4 and 11–5).

DIVISION OF THE PRIMITIVE ATRIUM.   Two localized proliferations of mesenchyme called *endocardial cushions* develop in the atrioventricular region of the heart (Fig. 11–5*A*). These cushions grow toward each other and fuse, dividing the atrioventricular canal into right and left atrioventricular (AV) canals (Fig. 11–5*B*). Before the **septum primum** fuses with these cushions, a communication exists between the right and left halves of the primitive atrium through the ostium primum initially and later through the *foramen secundum* and *foramen ovale* (Fig. 11–5*A* to *C*).

As the septum primum fuses with the endocardial cushions, obliterating the foramen primum, the superior part of the septum primum breaks down creating another opening called the *foramen secundum* (Fig. 11–5*B* to *D*). As this round foramen

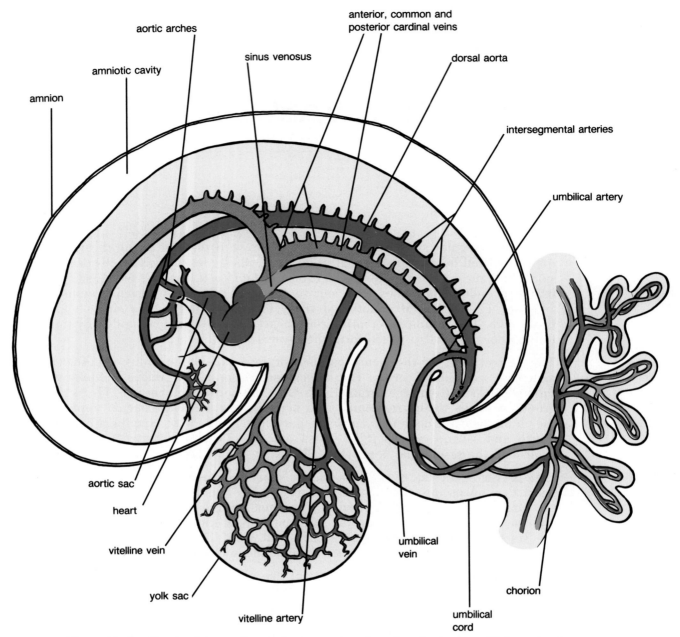

Figure 11–1.   Sketch of the cardiovascular system in a 4-week embryo, about 26 days, showing vessels of the left side only. The umbilical vein is shown in red because it carries well oxygenated blood and nutrients from the chorion (embryonic part of placenta) to the embryo. The umbilical arteries are colored blue to indicate that they are carrying poorly oxygenated blood and waste products to the chorion. See Figs. 4–3 to 4–5 and 11–10 for illustrations of the circulation through the placenta. (From Moore KL and Persaud TVN: *The Developing Human,* ed 5. Philadelphia, WB Saunders, 1993.)

develops, another sickle-shaped membranous fold, called the **septum secundum** grows into the atrium to the right of the septum primum (Fig. 11–5D to H). The septum secundum overlaps the foramen secundum, the opening in the septum primum. There is also an opening between the free edge of the septum secundum and the dorsal wall of the atrium, called the **foramen ovale** (Fig. 11–5E to H). By this stage, the remains of the septum primum has formed the flap-like valve of the foramen ovale.

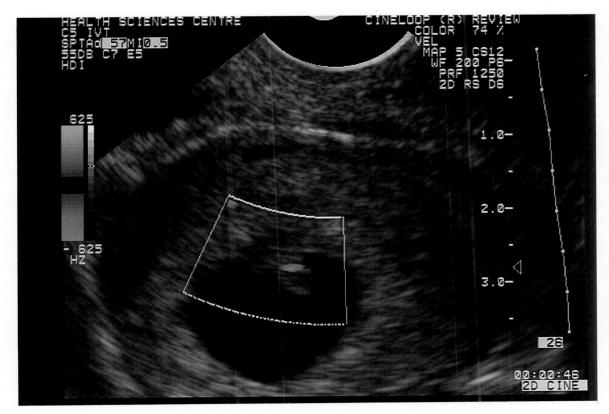

A

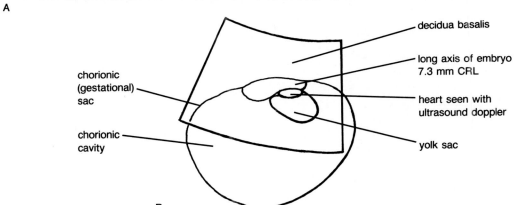

B

Figure 11-2. *A,* Sonogram of a 5-week embryo (7.2 mm) and its attached yolk sac within its chorionic (gestational) sac. The red pulsating heart of the embryo was visualized using Doppler ultrasound. (For a photograph of an embryo at this stage, see Fig. 2–16). *B,* Sketch of the sonogram for orientation and identification of structures. (Courtesy of Dr. E.A. Lyons, Professor of Radiology and Obstetrics and Gynecology and Head, Department of Radiology, Health Sciences Centre, University of Manitoba, Winnipeg, Manitoba, Canada.)

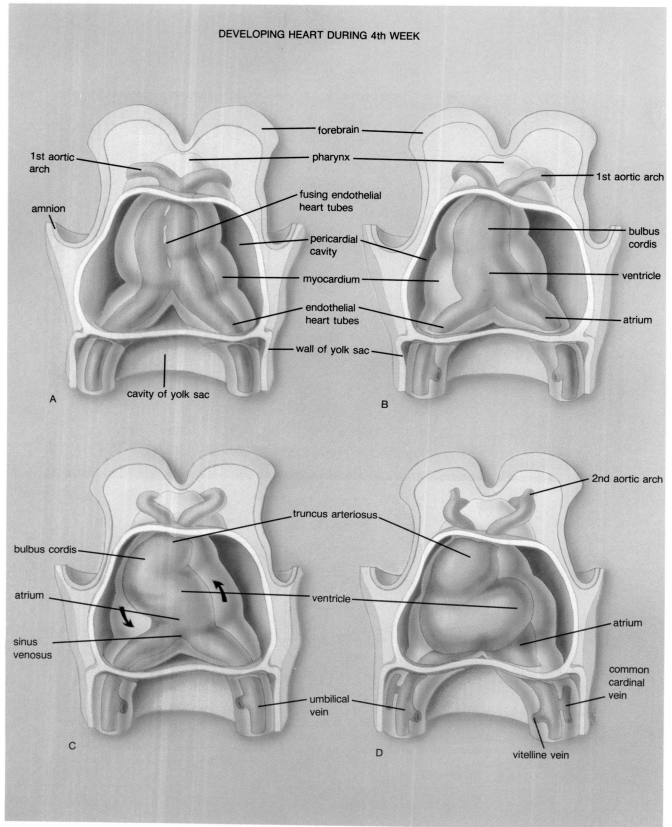

DEVELOPING HEART DURING 4th WEEK

Figure 11–3. Drawings of ventral views of the developing heart during the fourth week. Note that the endothelial heart tubes gradually fuse to form a single tubular heart. The fusion begins at the cranial ends of the tubes and extends caudally until a single tubular heart is formed. The endothelial heart tubes form the endocardium of the heart. They are derived from splanchnic mesenchyme (embryonic connective tissue), as is the myocardium or muscular wall of the heart. As the heart elongates, it bends upon itself, forming an S-shaped heart (D), and establishes its regional divisions.

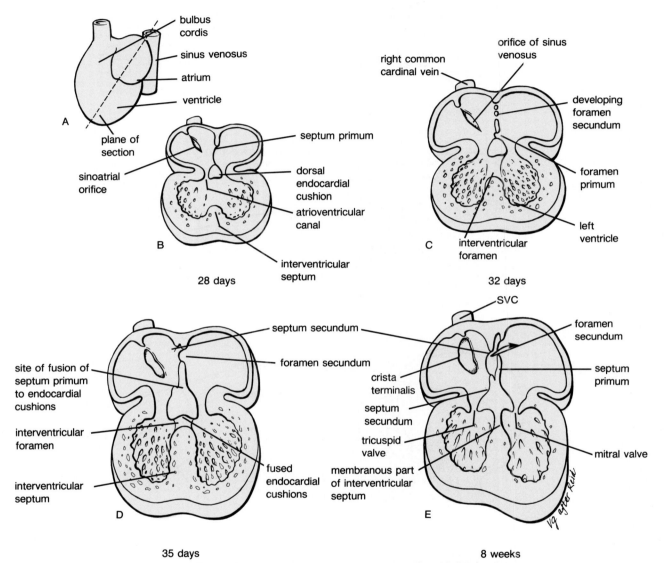

Figure 11–4. Drawings of the developing heart, showing partitioning of the atrioventricular canal, primitive atrium, and ventricle. *A,* Sketch showing the plane of the coronal sections. *B,* During the fourth week (about 28 days), showing the early appearance of the septum primum, interventricular septum, and dorsal endocardial cushion. *C,* Section of the heart (about 32 days), showing perforations in the dorsal part of the septum. *D,* Section of the heart (about 35 days) showing the foramen secundum. *E,* About eight weeks, showing the heart after it is partitioned into four chambers.

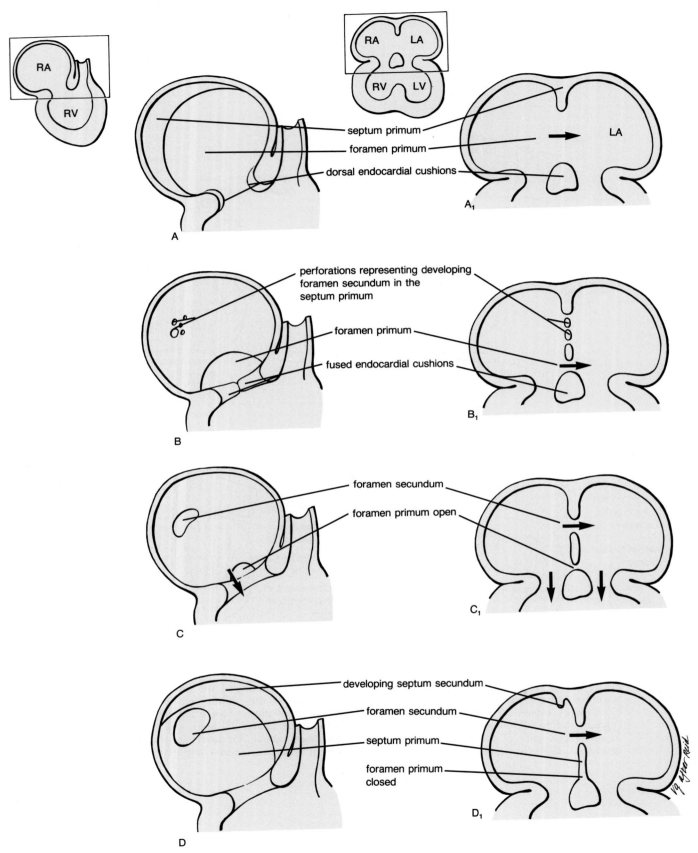

Figure 11–5. Diagrammatic sketches illustrating partitioning of the primordial atrium. A_1 to H_1 are coronal sections of the developing interatrial septum. Note that as the septum secundum grows, it overlaps the opening in the septum primum (foramen secundum). The valve-like nature of the foramen ovale is illustrated in G_1 and H_1. When pressure in the right atrium exceeds that in the left atrium, blood passes from the right to the left side of the heart (H_1). When the pressures are equal or higher in the left atrium, the septum primum closes the foramen ovale (G_1).

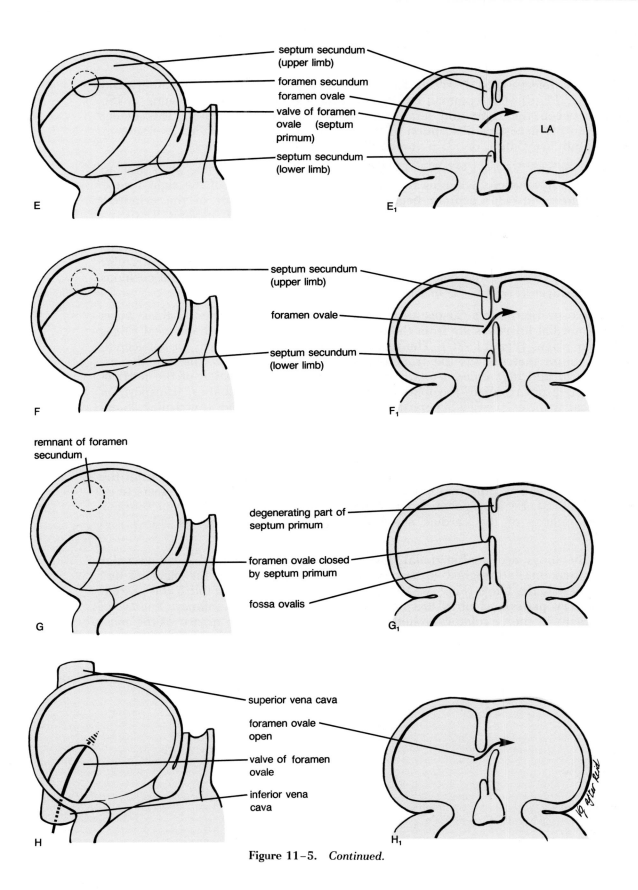

Figure 11–5. *Continued.*

The *conduction system of the heart* begins to develop in the fifth week and is well developed by the end of the eighth week. Recent experimental studies suggest that neural crest cells may contribute to the formation of the conducting system.

Atrial septal defects (ASDs) result from abnormal development of the interatrial septum (Fig. 11–6). The common defect is characterized by a large opening in the septum between the right and left atria **(persistent foramen ovale).** This defect results from (1) excessive absorption of the septum primum, (2) underdevelopment of the septum secundum, or (3) a combination of these abnormalities.

FORMATION OF THE VENTRICLES (Fig. 11–7). The primordial ventricle gives rise to most of the left ventricle, whereas the bulbus cordis forms most of the right ventricle. The *interventricular septum* begins as a ridge in the floor of the primitive ventricle (Fig. 11–7A) and slowly grows toward the endocardial cushions. Until the end of the seventh week, the future right and left ventricles communicate through a large **interventricular foramen** (see Fig. 11–7B). Closure of the interventricular foramen results in the formation of the membranous part of the interventricular septum. This part is derived from the fusion of tissue from the endocardial cushions and bulbar ridges (Fig. 11–7C to E).

PARTITIONING OF THE BULBUS CORDIS AND TRUNCUS ARTERIOSUS. Division of these parts of the primordial heart results from the development and fusion of the truncal ridges and bulbar ridges (Fig. 11–7C). The fused mesenchymal ridges form an aorticopulmonary septum that divides the truncus arteriosus and bulbus cordis into the *ascending aorta* and *pulmonary trunk*. Abnormalities in the formation of the aorticopulmonary septum result in the following major congenital anomalies: transposition of the great arteries (vessels), persistent truncus arteriosus, and ventricular septal defects. Ventricular septal defects (VSDs) are the most common congenital heart anomalies.

The critical period of heart development is from day 20 to day 50 after fertilization. Numerous critical events occur during cardiac development, and deviation from the normal pattern at any time may produce one or more congenital heart defects (e.g., ASDs and VSDs). Because partitioning of the primordial heart results from complex processes, defects of the cardiac septa are relatively common (Figs. 11–8 and 11–9).

Because the lungs are nonfunctional during prenatal life, the fetal cardiovascular system is structurally designed so that the blood is oxygenated in the placenta and largely bypasses the lungs (Fig. 11–10). The modifications that establish the postnatal circulatory pattern at birth are not abrupt but extend into infancy. Failure of these changes in the circulatory system to occur at birth results in two of the most common congenital abnormalities of the heart and great vessels: *patent foramen ovale* (Fig. 11–9) and *patent ductus arteriosus.*

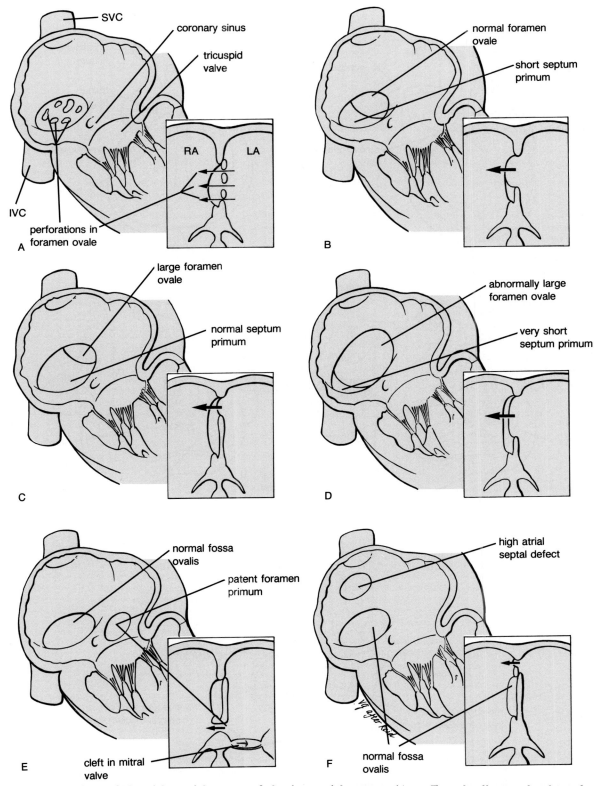

Figure 11–6. Drawings of the right atrial aspect of the interatrial septum (*A* to *F*) and adjacent sketches of coronal sections through the septum illustrating various types of atrial septal defect (ASD). *A,* Patent foramen ovale resulting from resorption of the septum primum in abnormal locations. *B,* Patent foramen ovale caused by excessive resorption of the septum primum, sometimes called the "short flap defect." *C,* Patent foramen ovale resulting from an abnormally large foramen ovale. *D,* Patent foramen ovale resulting from an abnormally large foramen ovale and excessive resportion of the septum primum. *E,* Endocardial cushion defect with primum-type atrial septal defect. *F,* Sinus venosus ASD due to abnormal absorption of the sinus venosus into the right atrium. In the sections *E* and *F,* note that the fossa ovalis has formed normally.

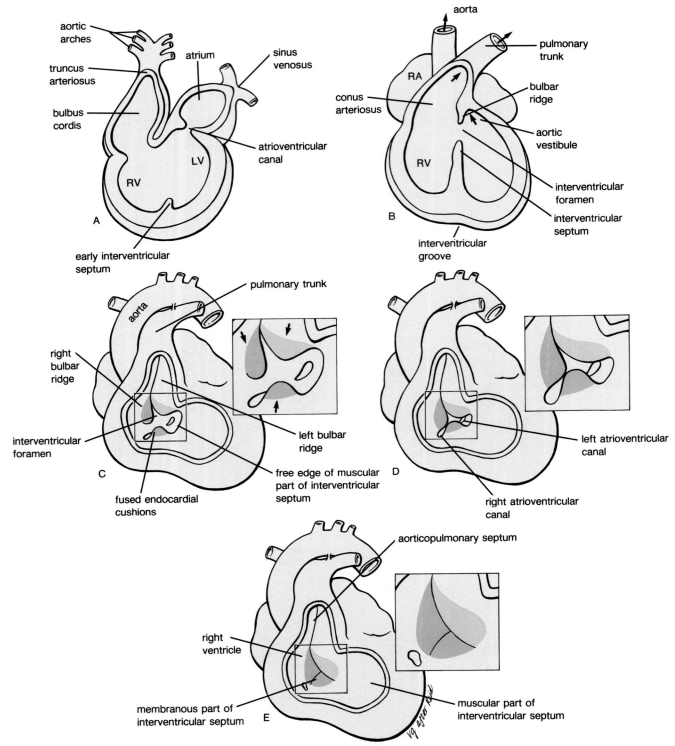

Figure 11-7. *A* and *B*, Sketches of the developing heart showing incorporation of the bulbus cordis into the ventricles and partitioning of the bulbus cordis and truncus arteriosus into the aorta and pulmonary trunk. *A*, Sagittal section at five weeks, showing the bulbus cordis as one of the five primordial chambers of the heart. *B*, Schematic coronal section at six weeks, after the bulbus cordis has been incorporated into the ventricles to form the conus arteriosus (infundibulum) of the right ventricle and the aortic vestibule of the left ventricle. *C* to *E*, Schematic drawings illustrating closure of the interventricular foramen and formation of the membranous part of the interventricular septum. The walls of the truncus arteriosus, bulbus cordis and right ventricle have been removed. *C*, Five weeks, showing the bulbar ridges and the fused endocardial cushions. *D*, Six weeks, showing how proliferation of subendocardial tissue diminishes the interventricular foramen. *E*, Seven weeks, showing the fused bulbar ridges and the membranous part of the interventricular septum formed by extensions of tissue from the right side of the endocardial cushions.

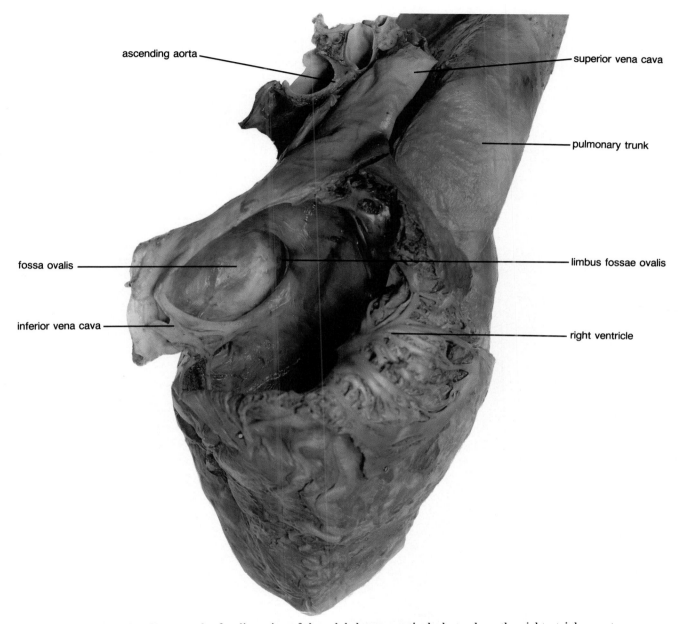

Figure 11-8. Photograph of a dissection of the adult heart, particularly to show the right atrial aspect of the interatrial septum. Observe the fossa ovalis and the limbus fossa ovalis. The floor of the fossa is formed by the septum primum, whereas the limbus fossa ovalis is formed by the free edge of the septum secundum (see Fig. 11–5G and G_1). Aeration of lungs at birth is associated with a dramatic fall in pulmonary vascular resistance and a marked increase in pulmonary flow. Due to the increased pulmonary blood flow, the pressure in the left atrium is raised above that in the right atrium. This increased left atrial pressure closes the foramen ovale by pressing the valve of the foramen ovale against the septum secundum (see Fig. 11–5G_1). This forms the fossa ovalis, a landmark of the interatrial septum.

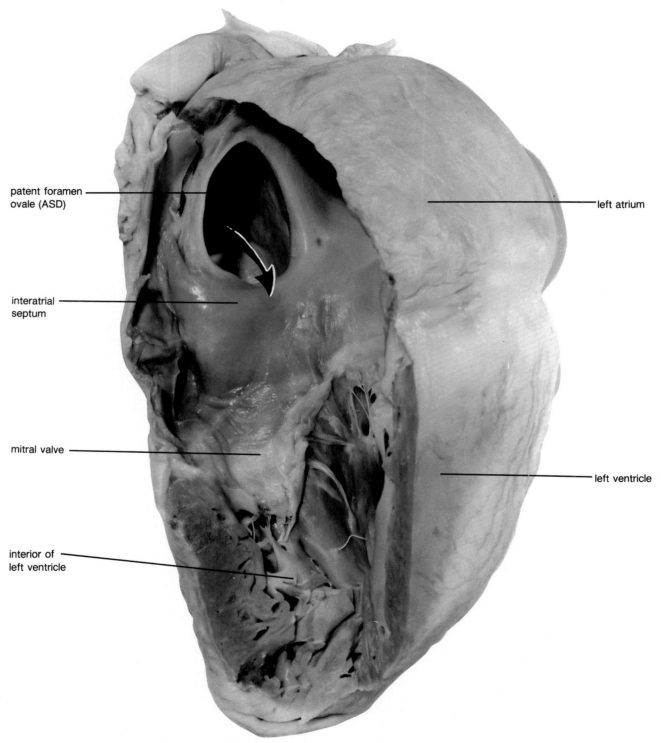

patent foramen ovale (ASD)

left atrium

interatrial septum

mitral valve

left ventricle

interior of left ventricle

Figure 11–9. Photograph of a dissection of an adult male heart with a large patent foramen ovale. The arrow passes through a large atrial septal defect (ASD) which resulted from an abnormally large foramen ovale and excessive resorption of the septum primum (see Fig. 11–6D). This is referred to as a secundum type ASD and is one of the most common types of congenital cardiac defect. The right ventricle and atrium are enlarged.

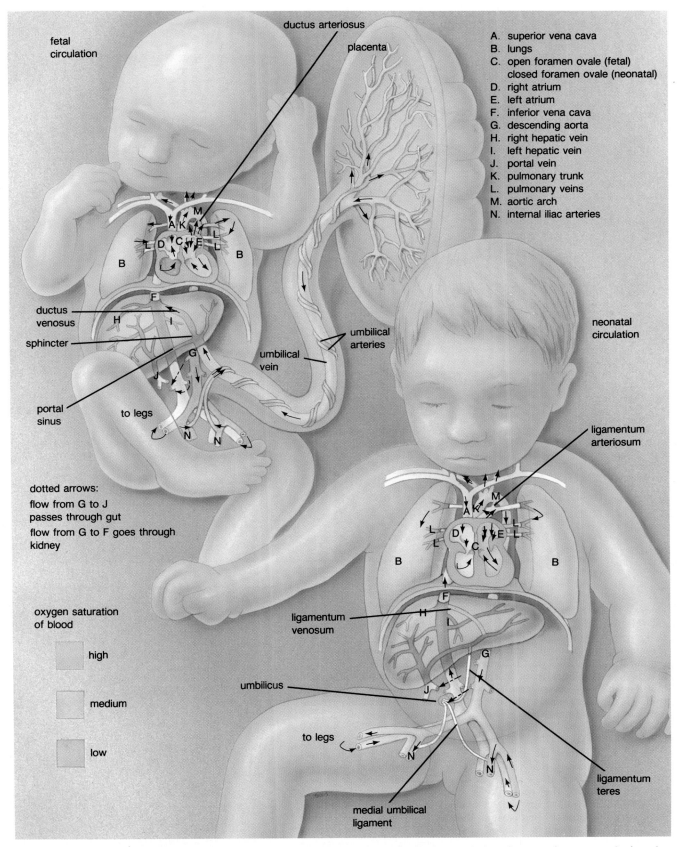

fetal circulation

ductus arteriosus

placenta

A. superior vena cava
B. lungs
C. open foramen ovale (fetal)
   closed foramen ovale (neonatal)
D. right atrium
E. left atrium
F. inferior vena cava
G. descending aorta
H. right hepatic vein
I. left hepatic vein
J. portal vein
K. pulmonary trunk
L. pulmonary veins
M. aortic arch
N. internal iliac arteries

ductus venosus

sphincter

portal sinus

to legs

dotted arrows:

flow from G to J passes through gut

flow from G to F goes through kidney

oxygen saturation of blood

high

medium

low

umbilical arteries

umbilical vein

neonatal circulation

ligamentum arteriosum

ligamentum venosum

umbilicus

medial umbilical ligament

to legs

ligamentum teres

Figure 11–10. Schematic illustrations showing the plan of the fetal circulation and the changes that occur during the neonatal period. The modifications that occur in the cardiovascular system result from the beginning of respiration and the cessation of placental blood flow.

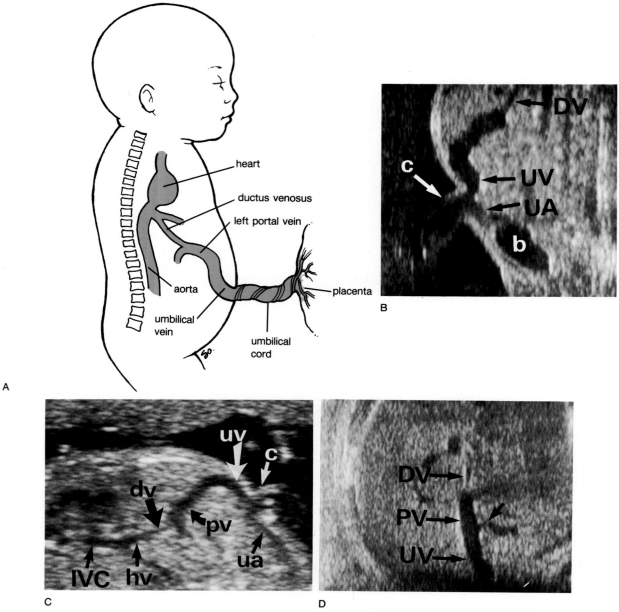

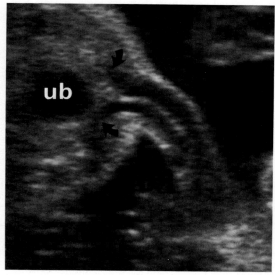

Figure 11–11. *A,* Schematic illustration of the course of the umbilical vein from the umbilical cord to the liver (see also Fig. 11–12*B*). *B,* Fetus with placental chorioangioma. The umbilical vein appears prominent. c, umbilical cord; b, bladder; UV, umbilical vein; UA, umbilical artery; DV, ductus venosus. *C,* Sagittal view of the fetal abdomen. c, Umbilical cord insertion; ua, umbilical artery. The umbilical vein (uv) courses cranially (cephalad) to the left portal vein (pv). The ductus venosus (dv) is a narrow channel that connects the left portal vein to the left hepatic vein (hv) or inferior vena cava (IVC). It shunts blood from the umbilical vein to the IVC, thereby bypassing the liver. *D,* This ultrasound scan shows the umbilical vein (UV) as it becomes the left portal vein (PV). The branch vessel *(arrow)* distinguishes this vessel (PV) from the umbilical vein. DV, ductus venosus (see also Fig. 11–12*B*). *E,* The umbilical cord insertion demonstrates the proximity of the distal umbilical arteries *(arrows)* to the wall of the urinary bladder (ub). The ductus venosus (DV) joins the inferior vena cava as shown in C. (From Goldstein RB, Callen PW: Ultrasound evaluation of the fetal thorax and abdomen. *In* Callen PW (ed): *Ultrasonography in Obstetrics and Gynecology,* ed 2. Philadelphia, WB Saunders, 1988).

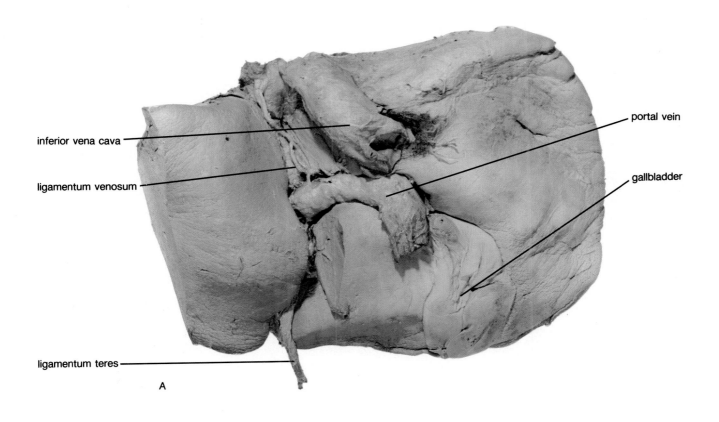

inferior vena cava

ligamentum venosum

ligamentum teres

A

portal vein

gallbladder

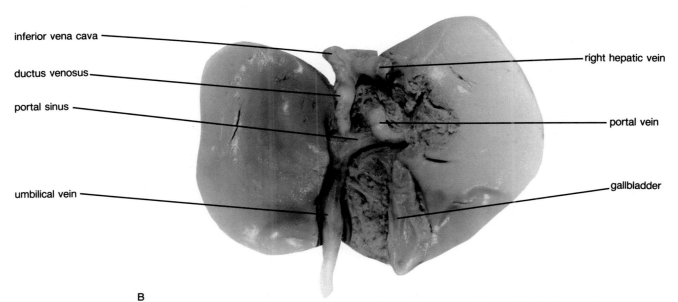

inferior vena cava

ductus venosus

portal sinus

umbilical vein

B

right hepatic vein

portal vein

gallbladder

Figure 11–12.   Photographs of dissections of the visceral surface of the liver. *A*, Adult. *B*, Fetus. Note that the umbilical vein is represented in the adult by the ligamentum teres and the ductus venosus by the ligamentum venosum (also see Fig. 11–10).

12

THE MUSCULOSKELETAL SYSTEM

Most parts of the muscular and skeletal systems, including the limbs, are derived from mesoderm (Figs. 12–1 to 12–3). The skeleton mainly develops from condensed mesenchyme (embryonic connective tissue), which undergoes chondrification to form hyaline cartilage models of the bones. Ossification centers appear in these models by the end of the embryonic period (eight weeks) and the bones ossify by *endochondral ossification* (Figs. 12–4 to 12–6). Some bones (e.g., the flat bones of the skull) develop by *intramembranous ossification.*

The **vertebral column and ribs** develop from sclerotomal cells that arise from the somites (Figs. 12–1 and 12–2; see also Fig. 2–6). Initially, the mesenchymal column retains traces of its segmental origin from the somites as the sclerotomal blocks are separated by less dense areas (Fig. 12–2). The **notochord** regresses in the area of the developing vertebral bodies, but it persists and enlarges in the region of the developing intervertebral discs. Here it gives rise to the *nucleus pulposus* of the disc, which is later surrounded by the circular fibers of the *anulus fibrosis.* The combination of these structures forms the *intervertebral disc.*

The **skull** develops from cells that are derived from paraxial mesoderm and the *neural crest.* The skull consists of a neurocranium and a viscerocranium, each of which has membranous and cartilaginous components. The *neurocranium* is divided into two parts: (1) a membranous part consisting of flat bones which surround the brain and form the calvaria (cranial vault), and (2) a cartilaginous part (chondrocranium), which forms the bones of the base of the skull (Fig. 12–7). The *viscerocranium* consists of the bones of the face and is formed mainly by the cartilages of the first two pairs of branchial or pharyngeal arches (Fig. 12–3; see also Fig. 7–4).

The **limb buds** appear toward the end of the fourth week as slight elevations of the ventrolateral body wall (Fig. 12–8; see also Fig. 2–11). The *apical ectodermal ridge* (AER), a thickening of ectoderm at the distal end of the limb bud, exerts an inductive influence on the mesenchyme in the limb buds that promotes growth and development of the limbs. The upper limb buds develop two days before the lower limb buds. The tissues of the limb buds are derived from three sources, the somatic layer of lateral mesoderm, the somitic mesoderm (Fig. 12–3A_1), and the ectoderm. The nerves grow into the limb buds during the fifth week (Fig. 12–3B). The upper and lower limbs rotate in opposite directions and to different degrees.

Most **skeletal muscle** is derived from the myotome regions of the somites (Fig. 12–3), but some head and neck muscles are derived from branchial or pharyngeal arch mesenchyme which is of neural crest origin (Chapter 7). Recent experimental studies suggest that the limb musculature develops from mesenchyme derived from the somites. Cardiac muscle and smooth muscle are mainly derived from splanchnic mesoderm.

Text continued on page 207

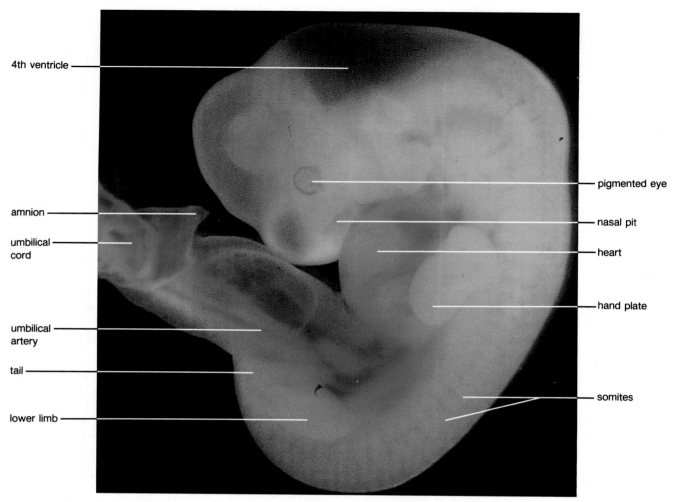

4th ventricle

amnion

umbilical cord

umbilical artery

tail

lower limb

pigmented eye

nasal pit

heart

hand plate

somites

Figure 12-1. Photograph of a lateral view of an embryo at Carnegie stage 15, about 36 days (see also Fig. 2-16). Mesenchymal models of the limb bones (not visible) have begun to form in a proximodistal sequence (i.e., the humerus appears before the forearm bones).

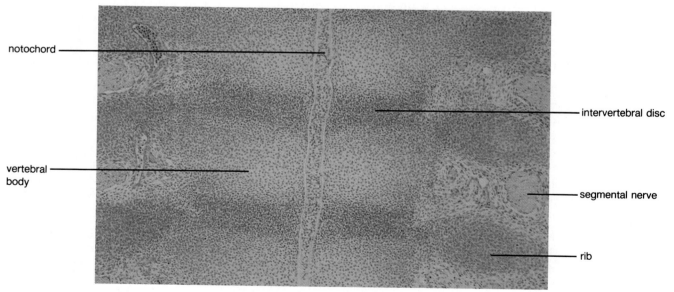

notochord

vertebral body

intervertebral disc

segmental nerve

rib

Figure 12-2. Coronal section of the axial region of an embryo at Carnegie stage 18, about 44 days. Observe the cartilaginous primordia of the vertebral bodies and ribs. Also observe the notochord in the center of the developing vertebrae. It will disappear except for the portion that forms the nucleus pulposus of the intervertebral disc. (From Nishimura H (ed): *Atlas of Human Prenatal Histology.* Tokyo, Igaku-Shoin, 1983.)

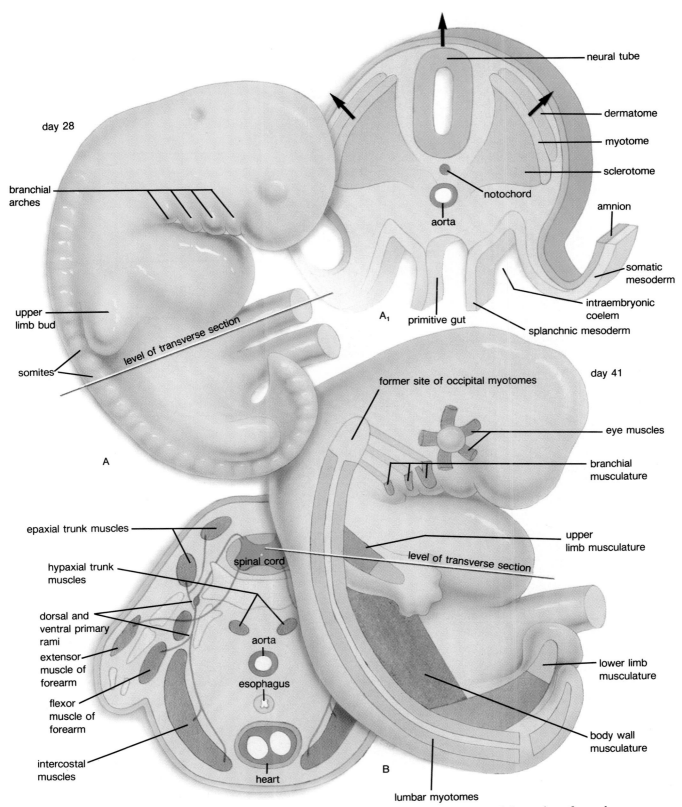

Figure 12–3. Drawings of embryos illustrating differentiation of the somites and formation of muscles. *A,* Embryo at 28 days. The *arrows* in A_1 indicate the directions of the somite remnants and the neural tube in relation to the notochord. *B,* Embryo at 41 days showing the muscle layers formed from the myotome regions of the somites. The limb muscles develop in situ from somatic mesoderm.

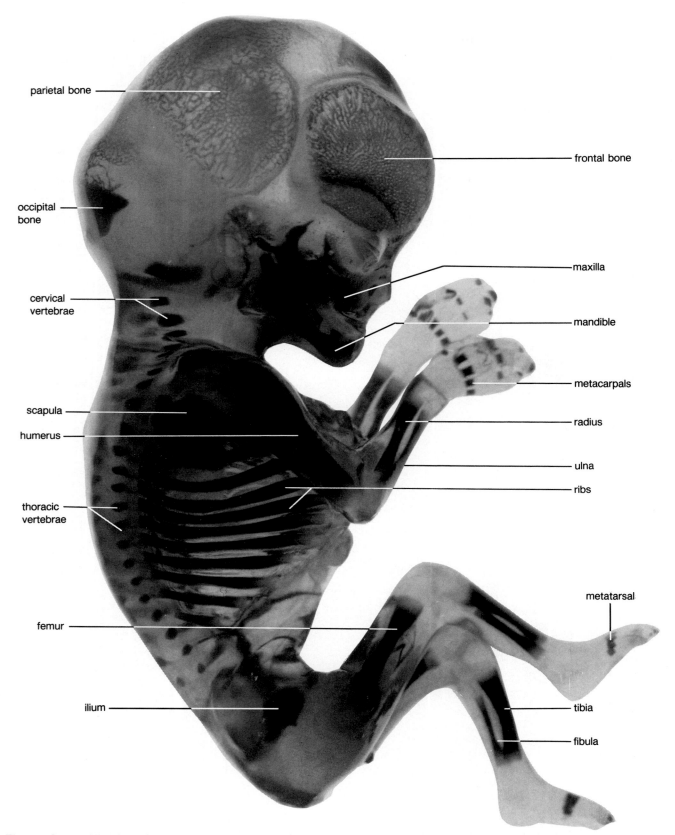

parietal bone

frontal bone

occipital bone

maxilla

cervical vertebrae

mandible

metacarpals

scapula

radius

humerus

ulna

ribs

thoracic vertebrae

femur

metatarsal

ilium

tibia

fibula

Figure 12–4.   Alizarin-stained and cleared 12-week human fetus. Observe the degree of progression of ossification from the primary centers of ossification, which is endochondral in the appendicular and axial parts of the skeleton except for most of the cranial bones (i.e., those that form the calvaria or cranial vault). Observe that the carpus and tarsus are wholly cartilaginous at this stage, as are the epiphyses of all long bones. (Courtesy of Dr. Gary Geddes, Lake Oswego, Oregon.)

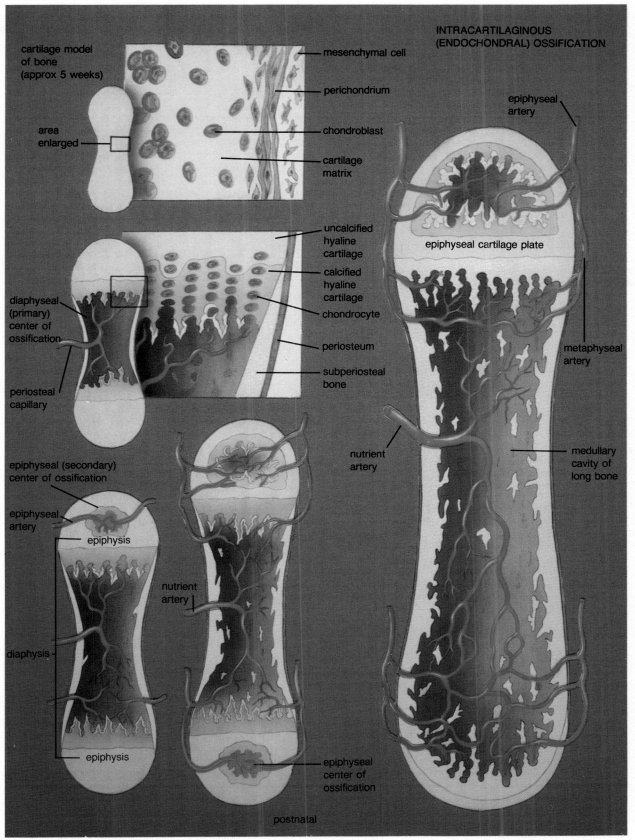

Figure 12-5. Schematic diagrams illustrating intracartilaginous or endochondral ossification and the development of a typical long bone. For details of endochondral ossification, see Cormack (1993).

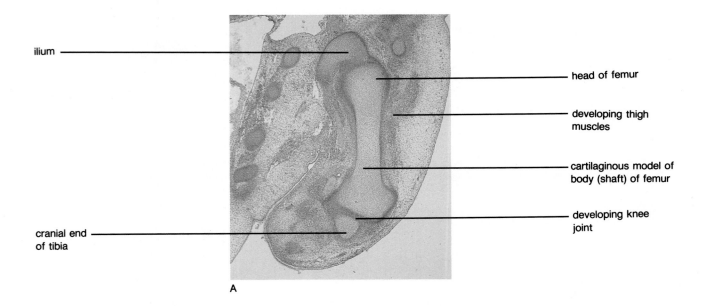

ilium

head of femur

developing thigh
muscles

cartilaginous model of
body (shaft) of femur

developing knee
joint

cranial end
of tibia

A

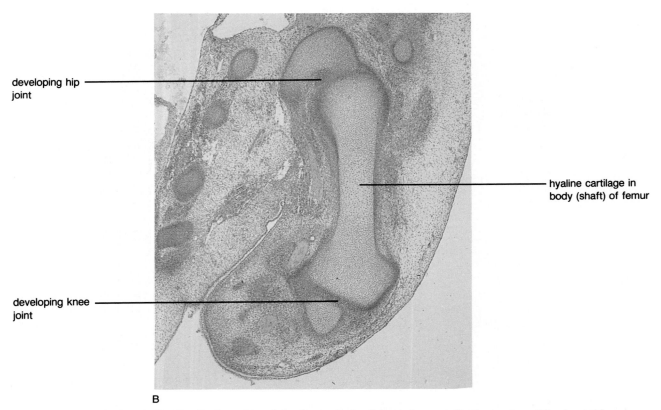

developing hip
joint

hyaline cartilage in
body (shaft) of femur

developing knee
joint

B

Figure 12-6. *A,* Longitudinal section of the lower limb of an embryo at Carnegie stage 19, about 48 days (×75). (See Fig. 2-21 for the appearance and size of an embryo at this stage.) Chondrification has begun in the bone and occurs in a proximodistal sequence. *B,* Higher magnification of this femur (×110).

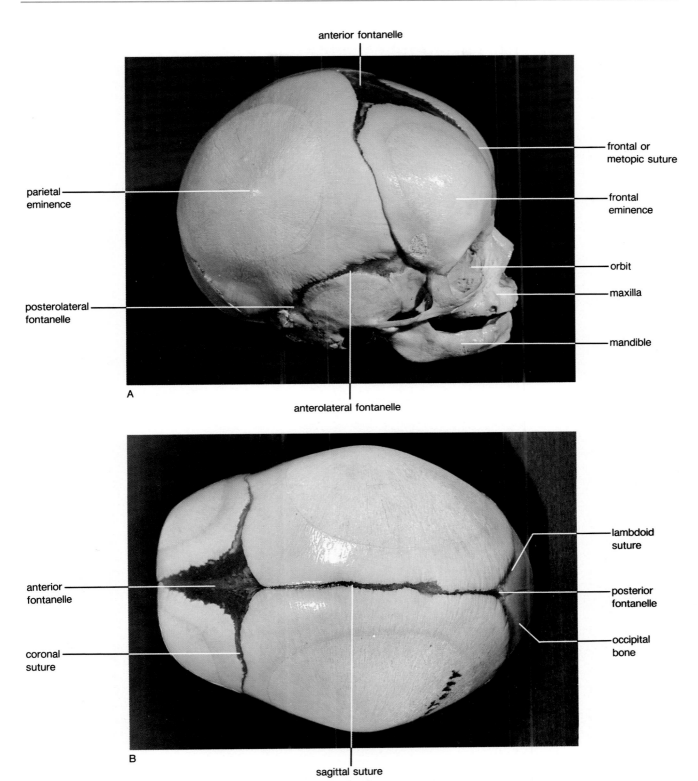

Figure 12–7. Photographs of a fetal skull showing the bones, fontanelles, and connecting sutures. *A,* Lateral view. *B,* Superior view. The posterior and anterolateral fontanelles disappear by growth of surrounding bones within two or three months after birth, but they remain as sutures for several years. The posterolateral fontanelles disappear in a similar manner by the end of the first year, and the anterior fontanelle by the end of the second year. The two halves of the frontal bone normally begin to fuse during the second year, and the frontal or metopic suture is often obliterated by the eighth year. The other sutures begin to disappear during adult life, but the times when the sutures close are subject to wide variation.

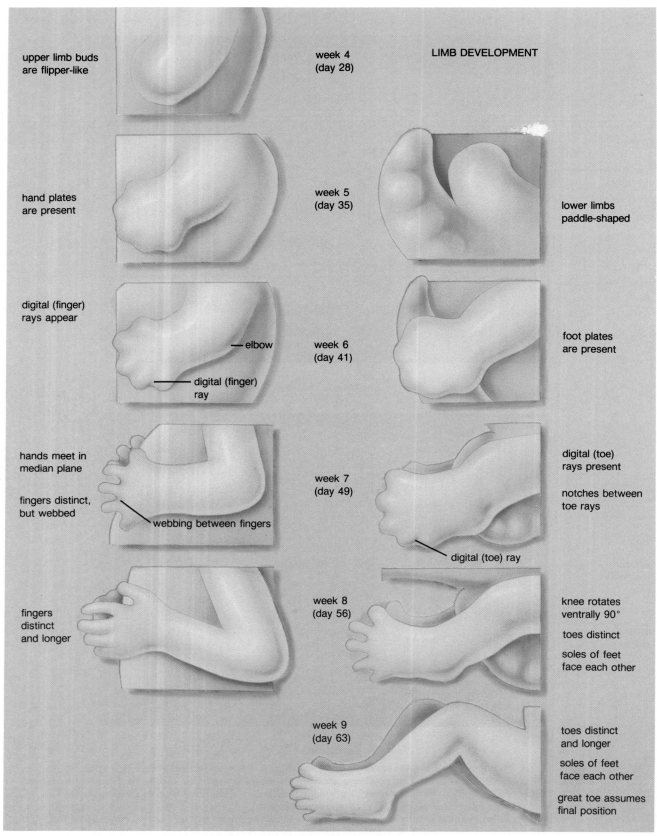

upper limb buds
are flipper-like

week 4
(day 28)

LIMB DEVELOPMENT

hand plates
are present

week 5
(day 35)

lower limbs
paddle-shaped

digital (finger)
rays appear

— elbow

week 6
(day 41)

— digital (finger)
ray

foot plates
are present

hands meet in
median plane

fingers distinct,
but webbed

webbing between fingers

week 7
(day 49)

digital (toe)
rays present

notches between
toe rays

digital (toe) ray

fingers
distinct
and longer

week 8
(day 56)

knee rotates
ventrally 90°

toes distinct

soles of feet
face each other

week 9
(day 63)

toes distinct
and longer

soles of feet
face each other

great toe assumes
final position

Figure 12–8. Drawings illustrating development of the limbs. The upper limb buds are visible by day 26 or 27; the lower limb buds appear two days later (see also Figs. 2–11 to 2–26). The stages of limb development are alike for the upper and lower limbs, except that development of the upper limbs precedes that of the lower limbs.

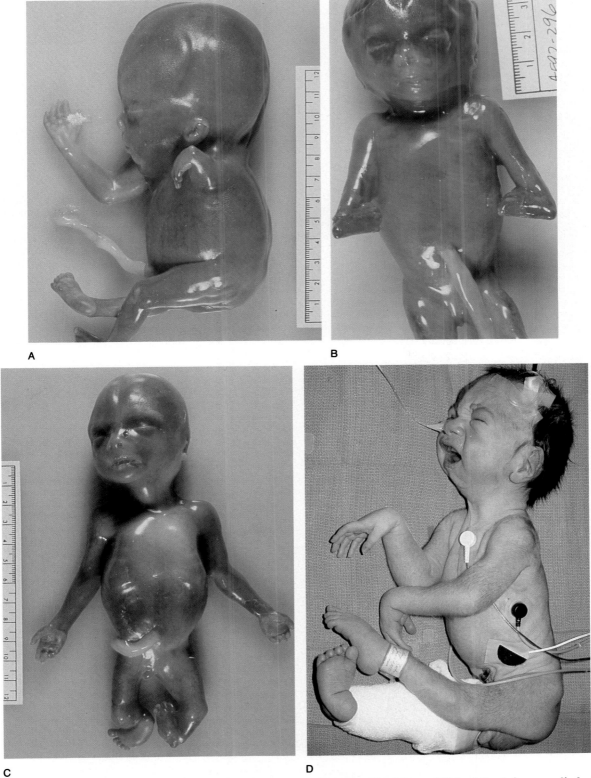

Figure 12–9. *A,* Female fetus (16 weeks) with a large head and meromelia (phocomelia) of the left upper limb. In the complete form, the hand arises directly from the trunk (i.e., the arm and forearm are absent). *B,* Absent radii in a 13.5-week female fetus. This anomaly may be associated with thrombocytopenia. *C,* Male fetus (16 weeks) with tibial aplasia on the right and hypoplasia on the left. *D,* Neonate with multiple joint contractures. Observe the elbows, knees, hips, and ankles (arthrogryposis). The common cause of this severe condition is decreased fetal activity due to neuromuscular deficiency. Also observe the micrognathia, i.e., small jaw. (*A, B,* and *C,* courtesy of Dr. D.K. Kalousek, Professor, Department of Pathology, University of British Columbia, Vancouver, B.C., Canada. *D,* courtesy of Dr. A.E. Chudley, Children's Centre, Winnipeg, Manitoba, Canada.)

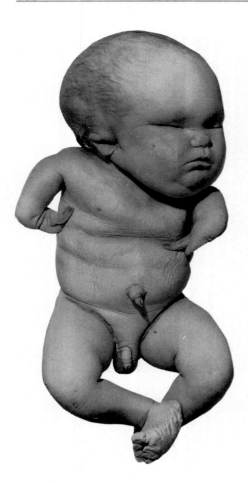

Figure 12–10. Near-term male fetus with a large head and low-set, malformed ears. There is also absence of the central digits of the hands resulting in split hands ("lobster claw anomaly"). These limb defects are usually autosomal dominant traits.

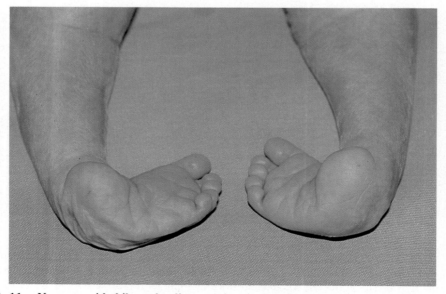

Figure 12–11. Neonate with bilateral talipes equinovarus deformities (clubfeet). This is the classic type with sharp and tight hyperextension and incurving of the feet.

Most **anomalies of the musculoskeletal system,** including those of the limbs, are caused by genetic factors; however, many congenital anomalies result from an interaction of genetic and environmental factors (multifactorial inheritance).

Limb defects vary greatly. In the most extreme form, one or more of the limbs are absent *(amelia).* More commonly, part of a limb is absent (e.g., a hand) producing a defect is known as *meromelia* (Fig. 12–9A). If there are extra digits (fingers or toes), the condition is called *polydactyly.* The extra digit is often nonfunctional due to inadequate muscular connections. Abnormal fusion of the digits is called *syndactyly.* Normally, the mesenchyme between the developing digit breaks down as they develop (see Figs. 2–22 to 2–25). Failure of the process to occur results in fusion of one or more fingers or toes. Failure of bones to develop also occurs (Fig. 12–9B and C). Lack of fetal movement (e.g., due to neuromuscular abnormalities) may result in abnormal development of joints (Fig. 12–9D). An abnormal cleft in the hands (Fig. 12–10) or feet results from aplasia of the central digits.

Clubfoot is a common anomaly, occurring about once in 1000 births. It is characterized by an abnormal position of the foot that prevents normal weight bearing (Fig. 12–11). In the most common type, *talipes equinovarus,* the sole of the foot is turned medially and inverted. This defect is often a solitary anomaly, but not infrequently it is associated with congenital dislocation of the hip, myelomeningocele (see Fig. 13–15), arthrogryposis (Fig. 12–9D), or other defects. Mild cases of clubfoot may be due to in utero postural-induced compression (positional deformation). Clubfoot is bilateral in 50 per cent of cases; the male to female ratio is about 2:1.

13

THE NERVOUS SYSTEM

The central nervous system (CNS) develops from a dorsal thickening of ectoderm known as the *neural plate* (Figs. 13–1A and B). This slipper-shaped plate appears around the middle of the third week and soon infolds to form a *neural groove* that has neural folds on each side (Figs. 13–1C and D and 13–2). When the *neural folds* fuse to form the *neural tube* during the middle of the fourth week (Figs. 13–1C to F and 13–3), some neuroectodermal cells are not included in it but remain between the neural tube and the surface ectoderm as the *neural crest* (Figs. 13–1E and 13–3).

Most of the **neural tube** becomes the spinal cord (Figs. 13–4 and 13–5). The cranial end of the neural tube forms the brain, consisting of the forebrain, midbrain, and hindbrain (Figs. 13–6 and 13–7). The forebrain gives rise to the cerebral hemispheres and diencephalon. The midbrain becomes the adult midbrain, and the hindbrain gives rise to the pons, cerebellum, and medulla oblongata. The remainder of the neural tube becomes the spinal cord. The lumen of the neural tube becomes the ventricles of the brain and the central canal of the spinal cord. The walls of the neural tube thicken due to proliferation of its neuroepithelial cells. These cells give rise to all nerve and macroglial cells in the central nervous system. The microglial cells differentiate from mononuclear leukocytes that penetrate the blood brain barrier and enter the central nervous system. Cells in the cranial, spinal, and autonomic ganglia are derived from the **neural crest** (Figs. 13–1E and 13–3). Schwann cells, which myelinate the axons external to the spinal cord, also arise from the neural crest. Similarly, most of the autonomic nervous system and all chromaffin tissue, including the suprarenal medulla, develop from neural crest cells.

Hydrocephalus (Fig. 13–8), a progressive increase in ventricular volume, is due to either a relative or complete obstruction of flow of cerebrospinal fluid (CSF) or, much less commonly, to overproduction of CSF. There are three types of congenital anomaly of the nervous system: (1) structural abnormalities resulting from abnormal organogenesis (e.g., **neural tube defects** (NTDs) resulting from abnormal development of the neural tube [Figs. 13–9 to 13–18]), (2) disturbances in the organization of the cells of the nervous system (e.g., due to the effects of high doses of radiation and severe malnutrition) that result in mental retardation, and (3) *errors of metabolism,* which are often inherited and can lead to severe mental retardation due to an accumulation of toxic substances (e.g., phenylketonuria) or to a deficiency of essential substances (e.g., congenital hypothyroidism).

Congenital anomalies of the central nervous system are common (about 3 per 1000 births). Defects in the closure of the neural tube (NTDs) account for most anomalies (e.g., **meningomyelocele** [Figs. 13–14 to 13–17]). The anomalies may be limited to the nervous system or they may include the overlying tissues (bone, muscle, and connective tissue). Gross congenital anomalies (e.g., meroanencephaly [Figs. 13–12 and 13–13]) are incompatible with life. Other severe defects (e.g., spina bifida with meningomyelocele) often cause functional disability, e.g., muscle paralysis of the lower limbs.

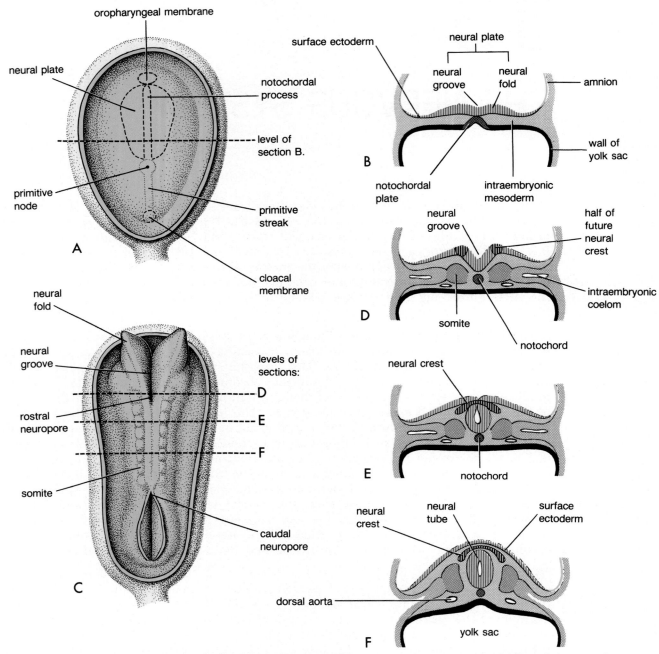

Figure 13-1. Drawings primarily illustrating formation of the neural crest and folding of the neural plate into the neural tube. *A,* Dorsal view of an embryo of about 18 days, exposed by removing the amnion. *B,* Transverse section of this embryo showing the neural plate and early development of the neural groove. The developing notochord is also shown (for details of its development, see Figs. 2–3D and 2–6D). *C,* Dorsal view of an embryo of about 22 days. The neural folds have fused opposite the somites but are widely spread out at both ends of the embryo. The rostral and caudal neuropores are indicated. Closure of the neural tube occurs initially in the region corresponding to the future junction of the brain and spinal cord. *D to F,* Transverse sections of this embryo at the levels shown in *C,* illustrating formation of the neural tube and its detachment from the surface ectoderm.

Mental retardation may result from chromosomal abnormalities arising during gametogenesis, from metabolic disorders, or from infections occurring during prenatal life (see Chapter 5). Various postnatal conditions (e.g., cerebral infection or trauma) may also cause abnormal mental development.

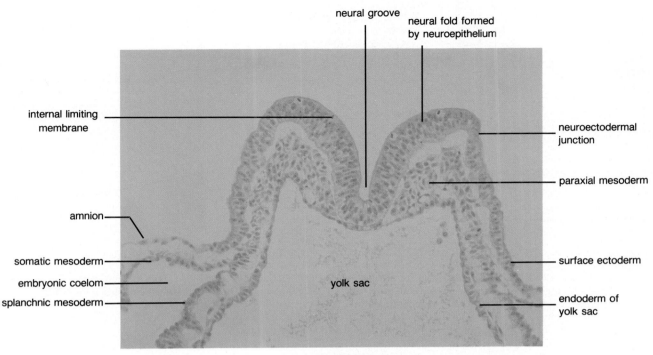

neural groove
neural fold formed
by neuroepithelium

internal limiting
membrane

neuroectodermal
junction

paraxial mesoderm

amnion

somatic mesoderm

embryonic coelom

splanchnic mesoderm

surface ectoderm

yolk sac

endoderm of
yolk sac

Figure 13-2. Transverse section of an embryo (×150) at Carnegie stage 10, about 21 days (see Fig. 2-7 for the appearance and size of an embryo at this stage). Observe the dividing cells in the neuroepithelium adjacent to the internal limiting membrane.

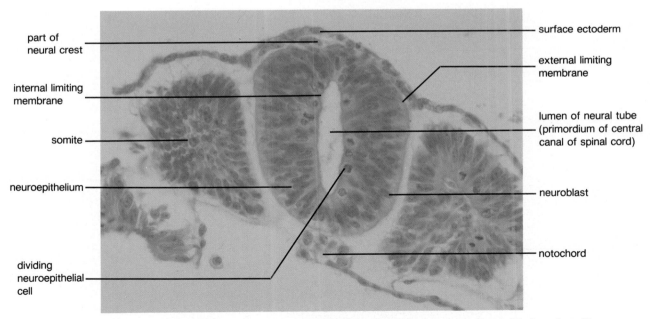

part of
neural crest

internal limiting
membrane

somite

neuroepithelium

dividing
neuroepithelial
cell

surface ectoderm

external limiting
membrane

lumen of neural tube
(primordium of central
canal of spinal cord)

neuroblast

notochord

Figure 13-3. Transverse section of an embryo (×300) at Carnegie stage 11, about 24 days (see Fig. 2-9 for the appearance and size of an embryo at this stage). Observe the neural tube, the primordium of the spinal cord in this region. At this stage, the neural tube is open at its cranial and caudal ends (Fig. 13-1*C*). Observe the dividing cells in the neuroepithelium adjacent to the internal limiting membrane. Mitotic cells are also visible in the somite on the left side. Neuroblasts (developing nerve cells) are visible near the external limiting membrane due to their large nuclei.

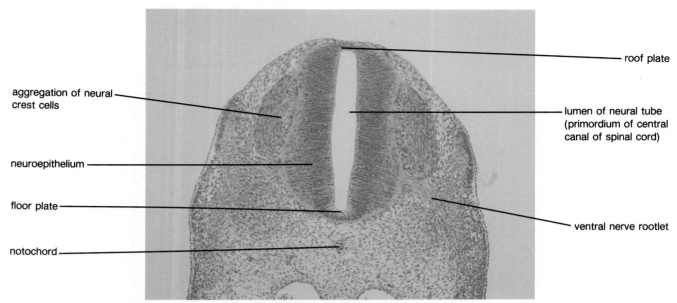

roof plate

aggregation of neural
crest cells

lumen of neural tube
(primordium of central
canal of spinal cord)

neuroepithelium

floor plate

ventral nerve rootlet

notochord

Figure 13-4. Transverse section of an embryo (×200) at Carnegie stage 13, about 28 days (see Fig. 2-12 for the appearance of an embryo at this stage). The central nervous system is a closed tube at this stage. Observe that the neuroepithelium is pseudostratified (due to the developing nerve cells at this stage). Aggregations of neural crest cells are located at the sides of the neural tube where they will differentiate into the ganglion cells of the spinal (dorsal root) ganglia.

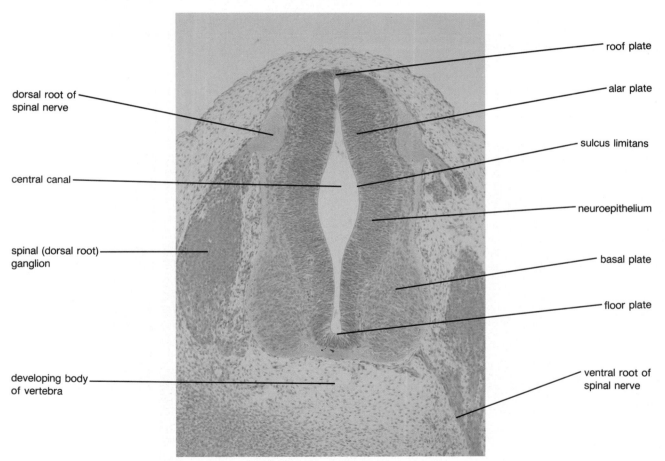

roof plate

alar plate

dorsal root of
spinal nerve

sulcus limitans

central canal

neuroepithelium

spinal (dorsal root)
ganglion

basal plate

floor plate

developing body
of vertebra

ventral root of
spinal nerve

Figure 13-5. Transverse section of an embryo (×100) at Carnegie stage 16, about 40 days (see Fig. 2-17 for the appearance and size of an embryo at this stage). The ventral root of the spinal nerve is composed of nerve fibers arising from neuroblasts (developing nerve cells) in the basal plate (developing ventral horn of the spinal cord), whereas the dorsal root is formed by nerve processes arising from neuroblasts in the spinal (dorsal root) ganglion.

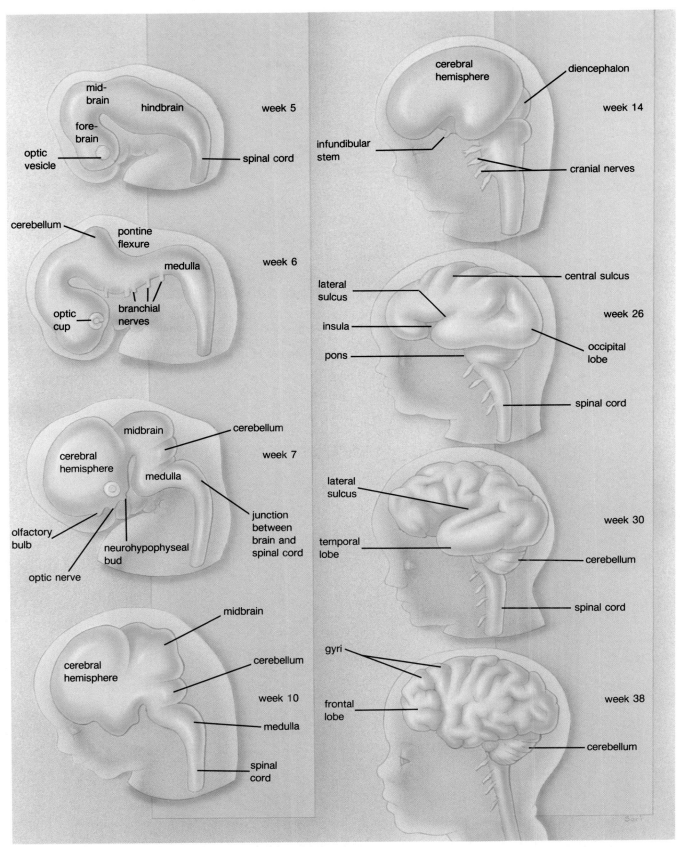

Figure 13–6. Series of drawings showing the developing brain and spinal cord at the ages indicated. They also demonstrate the changes in size and development of the sulci and gyri of the cerebral hemispheres.

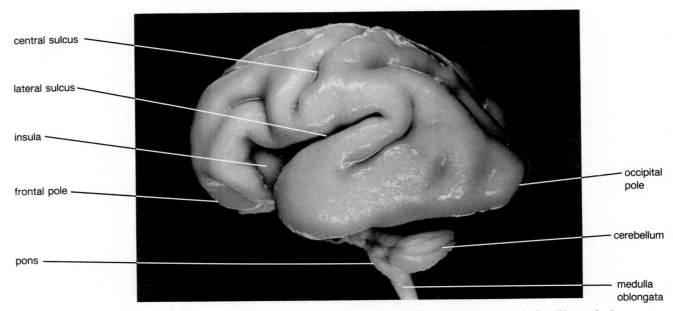

central sulcus

lateral sulcus

insula

frontal pole

pons

occipital pole

cerebellum

medulla oblongata

Figure 13–7.   Photograph of a lateral view of the brain of a stillborn fetus (25 weeks). See Figure 3–6 for the appearance of a fetus at this stage. (From Nishimura H, Semba R, Tanimura T, Tanaka O: *Prenatal Development of the Human with Special Reference to Craniofacial Structures: An Atlas.* US Department of Health, Education, and Welfare, National Institutes of Health, Bethesda, 1977.)

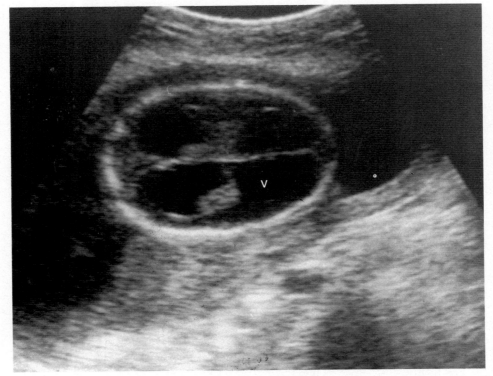

Figure 13–8.   Transverse axial sonogram of a 17-week gestation (15-week fetus) demonstrating hydrocephalus. Observe the enlarged ventricles (V) of the brain. This condition is usually due to a relative or complete obstruction of flow of cerebrospinal fluid (CSF), e.g., in the cerebral aqueduct. (Courtesy of Dr. Lyndon M. Hill, Director of Ultrasound, Magee-Women's Hospital, Pittsburgh, PA.)

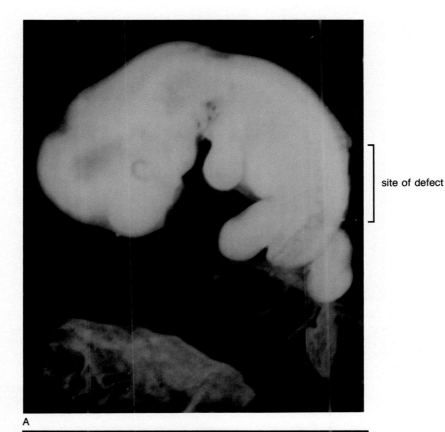

A

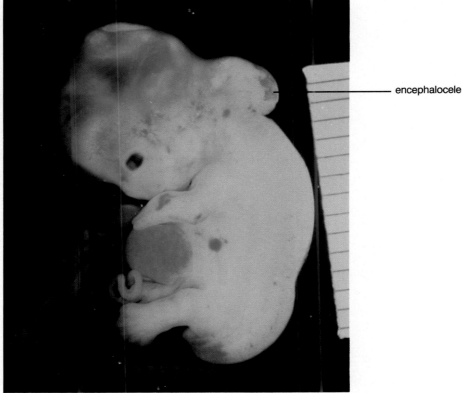

B

site of defect

encephalocele

Figure 13-9. *A,* Photograph of an embryo at Carnegie stage 16, about 38 days, with a defect in the lumbosacral area (see Fig. 2-17 for the appearance of a normal embryo at this stage). The abnormal embryo shown above had the following chromosome constitution: 70,XXY,+18. *B,* Photograph of an abnormal female embryo at Carnegie stage 19, about 45 days (see Fig. 2-21 for the appearance and size of a normal embryo at this stage). This embryo has an occipital encephalocele. (Courtesy of Dr. D.K. Kalousek, Professor, Department of Pathology, University of British Columbia, Vancouver, B.C., Canada.)

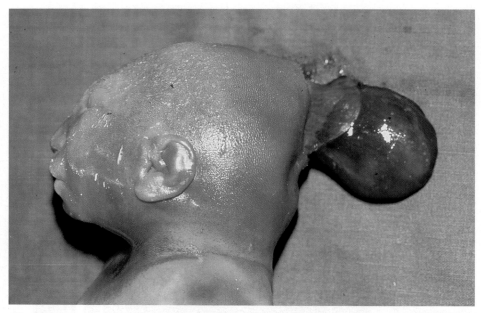

Figure 13–10. Photograph of an aborted fetus (about 16 weeks) with an occipital encephalocele consisting of a protrusion of the occipital lobe of the brain that is covered with cranial meninges. The ear is abnormally large and low set. (Courtesy of Dr. A.E. Chudley, Children's Centre, Winnipeg, Manitoba, Canada.)

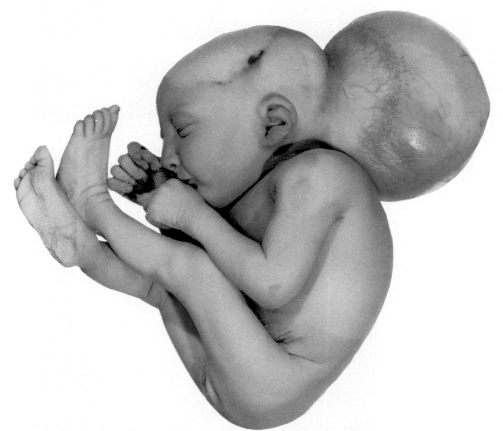

Figure 13–11. Photograph of a female neonate with a large meningoencephalocele in the occipital area due to a large defect in the occipital bone. It consists of a protrusion of the occipital lobe of the brain that is covered with cranial meninges and skin. (Courtesy of Dr. Dwight Parkinson, Children's Centre, Winnipeg, Manitoba, Canada.)

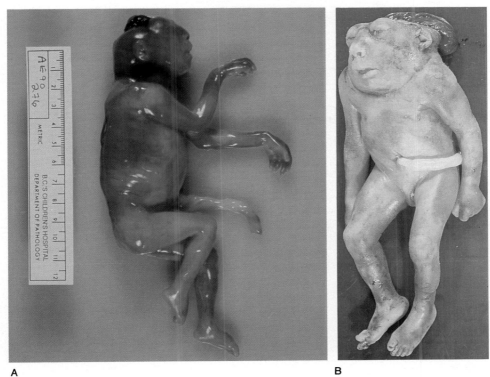

Figure 13-12. *A*, Photograph of a female fetus (16 weeks) with meroanencephaly or anencephaly. The remnant of the brain (hindbrain) appears as a spongy, vascular mass. *B*, Stillborn infant with meroanencephaly. Due to the absence of most of the brain, these infants do not survive. This is the most common of the open neural tube defects and the most common defect affecting the CNS. It shows a clear female predominance with a female to male ratio of 4:1. This severe defect results from failure of the rostral neuropore to close at the end of the fourth week. (*A*, Courtesy of Dr. D.K. Kalousek, Professor, Department of Pathology, University of British Columbia, Vancouver, B.C., Canada. *B*, Courtesy of Dr. A.E. Chudley, Children's Centre, Winnipeg, Manitoba, Canada.)

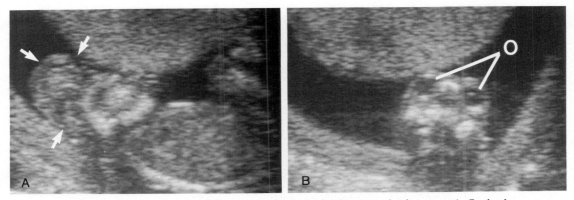

Figure 13-13. Meroanencephaly, or anencephaly, early in the second trimester. *A*, Sagittal sonogram demonstrating a large mass of angiomatous stroma *(arrows)* cephalad to the skull base. *B*, The coronal image of the face demonstrates the symmetric absence of the calvaria superior to the orbits (O), thus confirming the diagnosis of meroanencephaly. Even though this anomaly is often called anencephaly (without a brain), there is always functioning neural tissue present. For this reason, the term meroanencephaly (part brain) describes the anomaly better. The calvaria (cranial vault) is always absent (From Filly RA: Ultrasound evaluation of the fetal neural axis. *In* Callen PW (ed): *Ultrasonography In Obstetrics and Gynecology,* ed 2. Philadelphia, WB Saunders, 1988.)

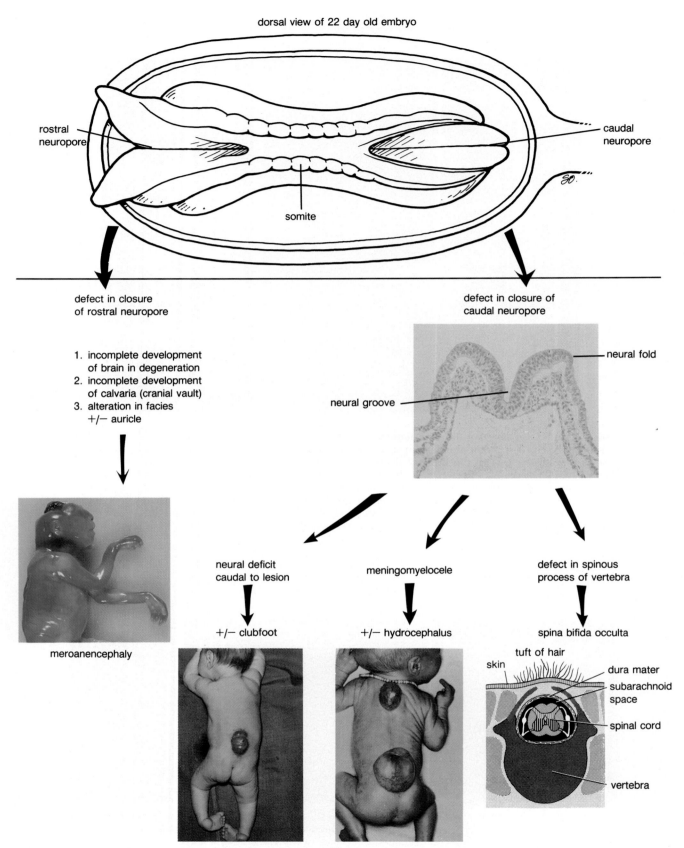

dorsal view of 22 day old embryo

rostral neuropore

caudal neuropore

somite

defect in closure of rostral neuropore

defect in closure of caudal neuropore

neural fold

neural groove

1. incomplete development of brain in degeneration
2. incomplete development of calvaria (cranial vault)
3. alteration in facies +/− auricle

neural deficit caudal to lesion

meningomyelocele

defect in spinous process of vertebra

+/− clubfoot

+/− hydrocephalus

spina bifida occulta

meroanencephaly

tuft of hair

skin

dura mater

subarachnoid space

spinal cord

vertebra

Figure 13–14. Schematic drawings and photographs illustrating and explaining the embryologic basis of neural tube defects (NTDs), such as meroanencephaly (anencephaly) and spina bifida with meningomyelocele. Meroanencephaly is due to defective closure of the rostral neuropore and meningomyelocele is due to defective closure of the caudal neuropore (Modified from Jones KL: *Smith's Recognizable Patterns of Human Malformations,* ed 4. Philadelphia, WB Saunders, 1988. Photograph of clubfoot is courtesy of Dr. Dwight Parkinson, Children's Centre, Winnipeg, Manitoba, Canada.)

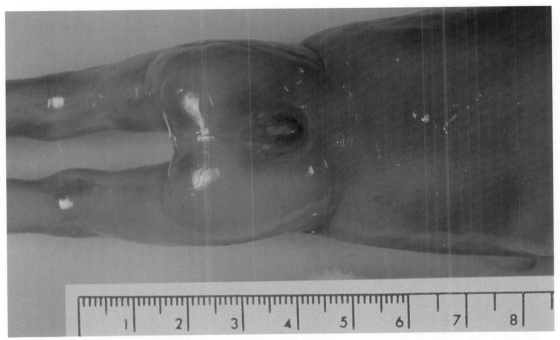

Figure 13–15. Photograph of the back of a 16.5-week female fetus with a lumbosacral meningomyelocele. A defect in the vertebral (neural) arches of the lower lumbar and upper sacral vertebrae resulted in protrusion of the meninges and defective development of the spinal cord. Meningomyeloceles are often accompanied by a marked neurological deficit inferior to the protruding sac (e.g., paralysis of the lower limbs and sphincter paralysis of the urinary bladder). These defects may be covered by skin or a thin, easily ruptured membrane as in this case. (Courtesy of Dr. D.K. Kalousek, Professor, Department of Pathology, University of British Columbia, Vancouver, B.C., Canada.)

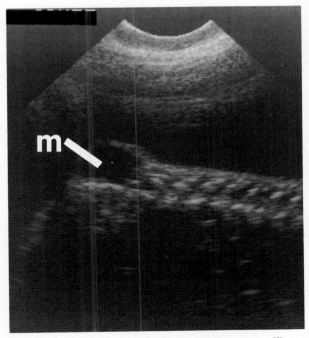

Figure 13–16. Ultrasound scan of a 14-week-old fetus, showing a cyst-like protrusion representing a meningomyelocele (m) in the sacral region of the vertebral column. The well formed vertebral (neural) arches of the vertebrae superior to the neural tube defect are clearly visible. (Courtesy of Dr. Lyndon, M. Hill, Director of Ultrasound, Magee-Women's Hospital, Pittsburgh, PA.)

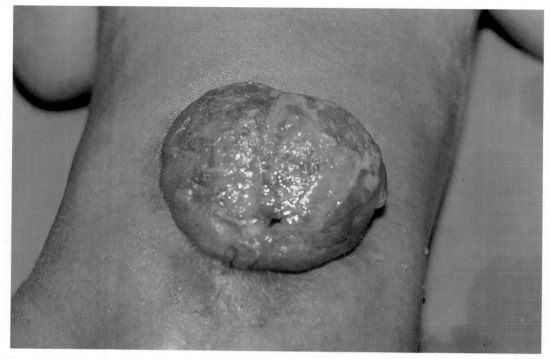

Figure 13-17. Photograph of the back of a neonate with a large lumbar meningomyelocele. The neural tube defect (NTD) was covered with a thin membrane. These defects may occur anywhere along the vertebral column, but they are most common in the lumbar region. For the embryologic basis of the NTD, see Figure 13-14. (Courtesy of Dr. A.E. Chudley, Children's Centre, Winnipeg, Manitoba, Canada).

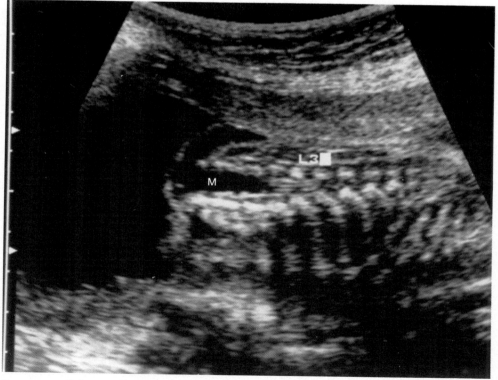

Figure 13-18. Sonogram of the caudal end of a 20-week fetus (22 weeks' gestation) showing myelorachischisis of the lower lumbar region of the vertebral column, distal to L3 vertebra. This defect resulted in a meningomyelocele (M) of the spinal cord. (Courtesy of Dr. Lyndon Hill, Director of Ultrasound, Magee-Women's Hospital, Pittsburgh, Pennsylvania).

14

THE EYE AND EAR

These special sense organs begin to develop during the fourth week. The eyes and ears are very sensitive to the teratogenic effects of infectious agents (e.g., cytomegalovirus and rubella virus; see Table 5-3). The most serious defects result from disturbances during the fourth to sixth weeks of development, but defects of sight and hearing may result from infection of tissues and organs by certain microorganisms during the fetal period (e.g., rubella virus and *Treponema pallidum*, the microorganism that causes syphilis).

THE EYE

The first indication of the eye is the *optic sulcus,* which forms at the beginning of the fourth week. This groove soon deepens to form a hollow *optic vesicle* that projects laterally from the forebrain (see Fig. 13-6). The optic vesicle contacts the surface ectoderm and induces development of the *lens placode* (see Fig. 2-11), the primordium of the lens. As the lens placode invaginates to form a *lens pit* and a *lens vesicle* (Figs. 14-1 and 14-3), the optic vesicle invaginates to form an **optic cup.** The retina forms from the two layers of the optic cup.

The **retina,** the optic nerve fibers, the muscles of the iris, and the epithelium of the iris and ciliary body are derived from the *neuroectoderm* of the forebrain (Figs. 14-1 to 14-5). The *surface ectoderm* gives rise to the lens and the epithelium of the lacrimal glands, eyelids, conjunctiva, and cornea. The head mesenchyme and the neural crest give rise to the eye muscles, except those of the iris, and to all connective and vascular tissues of the cornea, iris, ciliary body, choroid, and sclera. The sphincter and dilator muscles of the iris develop from the ectoderm at the rim of the optic cup.

There are many *ocular anomalies* but most of them are uncommon (Fig. 14-6). Most anomalies are caused by defective closure of the optic fissure (Fig. 14-3*B*) during the sixth week (e.g., coloboma of the iris). *Congenital cataract* and **glaucoma** may result from intrauterine infections (e.g., rubella virus [see Fig. 5-12]), but most congenital cataracts are inherited.

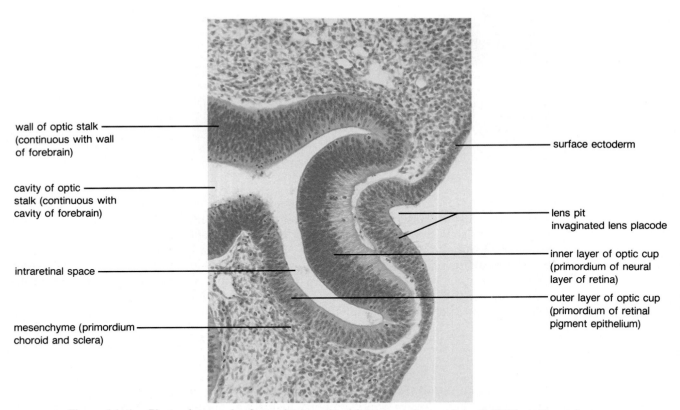

wall of optic stalk
(continuous with wall
of forebrain)

cavity of optic
stalk (continuous with
cavity of forebrain)

intraretinal space

mesenchyme (primordium
choroid and sclera)

surface ectoderm

lens pit
invaginated lens placode

inner layer of optic cup
(primordium of neural
layer of retina)

outer layer of optic cup
(primordium of retinal
pigment epithelium)

Figure 14–1. Photomicrograph of a sagittal section of the eye of an embryo (×200) at Carnegie stage 14, about 32 days. (See Fig. 2–15 for the external appearance and size of an embryo at this stage). Observe the primordium of the lens (invaginated lens placode), the walls of the optic cup (primordium of the retina), and the optic stalk (primordium of the optic nerve).

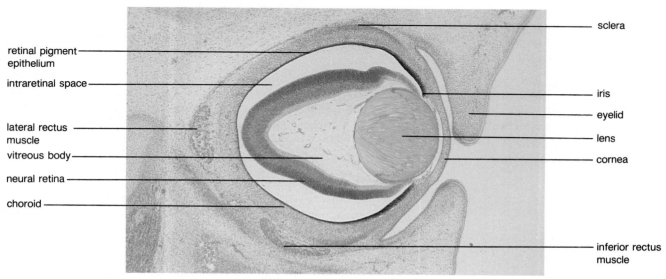

retinal pigment
epithelium

intraretinal space

lateral rectus
muscle

vitreous body

neural retina

choroid

sclera

iris

eyelid

lens

cornea

inferior rectus
muscle

Figure 14–2. Photomicrograph of a sagittal section of the eye of an embryo (×50) at Carnegie stage 23, about 56 days. (See Fig. 2–25 for the external appearance and size of an embryo at this stage). Observe the neural retina and the retinal pigment epithelium.

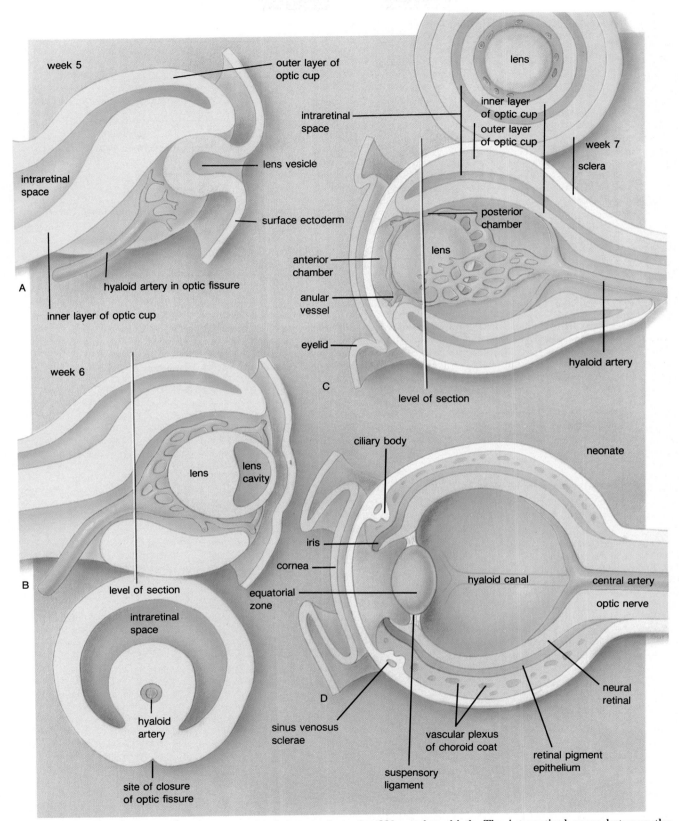

Figure 14-3. Drawings showing development of the eye from the fifth week to birth. The intraretinal space between the inner (primordium of neural retina) and outer (primordium of the retinal pigment epithelium) layers of the optic cup disappears as the eye develops. Trauma may separate the layers of the retina in this area. The hyaloid artery supplies the developing lens but most of it disappears. Its proximal part forms the central artery of the retina. The hyaloid canal in the vitreous body (shown in *D*) indicates the former site of the distal part of the hyaloid artery.

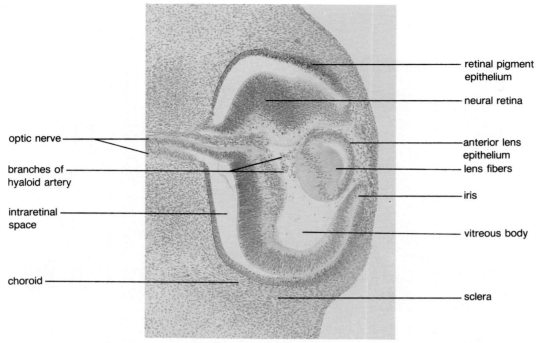

Figure 14-4. Photomicrograph of a sagittal section of the eye of an embryo (×100) at Carnegie stage 18, about 44 days. (See Fig. 2-20 for the external appearance and size of an embryo at this stage). Observe that it is the posterior wall of the lens vesicle that forms the lens fibers. The anterior wall does not change appreciably as it becomes the anterior lens epithelium. (From Nishimura H (ed): *Atlas of Human Prenatal Histology*. Igaku-Shoin, Tokyo, 1983).

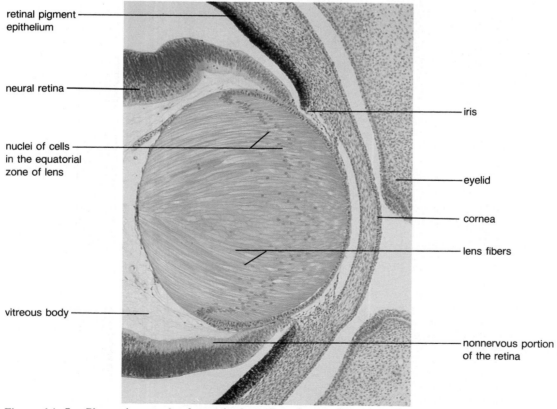

Figure 14-5. Photomicrograph of a sagittal section of a portion of the developing eye of an embryo (×280) at Carnegie stage 23, about 56 days. Observe that the lens fibers have elongated and obliterated the cavity of the lens vesicle. Note that the inner layer of the optic cup has thickened greatly to form the neural retina and that the outer layer is heavily pigmented (retinal pigment epithelium).

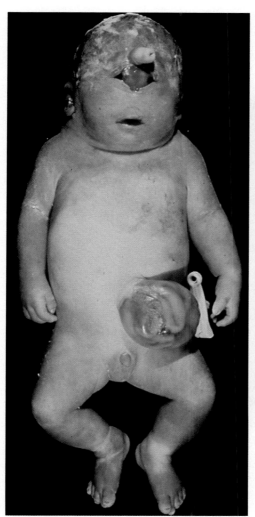

A

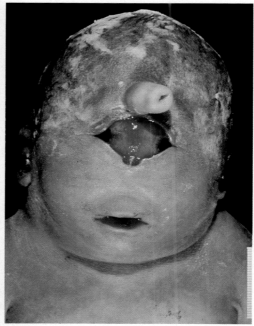

B

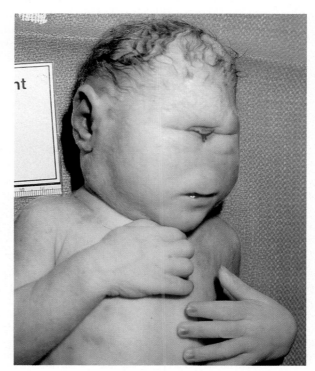

C

Figure 14-6. *A* and *B*, Male neonate with cyclopia (synoph-thalmia) and omphalocele (herniation of the intestines into the proximal part of the umbilical cord). Cyclopia (fusion of the eyes) is a severe, uncommon anomaly of the face and eye asso-ciated with a proboscis-like appendage located superior to the eye. Several facial bones are absent, e.g., nasal bones and eth-moids. *C*, Cyclopia in a neonate with absence of a proboscis. This condition and the one shown in *A* and *B* are due to holo-prosencephaly (failure of the forebrain to divide into cerebral hemispheres). This severe anomaly results from faulty interac-tion between the notochord and the neuroectoderm during the fourth week of development. These infants usually die during the neonatal period due to the presence of other major anoma-lies, e.g., of the forebrain. (*A* and *B*, courtesy of Dr. Susan Phillips, Department of Pathology, Health Sciences Centre, Win-nipeg, Manitoba, Canada. *C*, courtesy of Dr. A.E. Chudley, Chil-dren's Centre, Winnipeg, Manitoba, Canada.)

THE EAR

The surface ectoderm gives rise to the *otic vesicle* during the fourth week (Figs. 14–7 to 14–9). It develops into the membranous labyrinth of the internal ear. The otic vesicle divides into: (1) a dorsal utricular portion, which gives rise to the utricle, semicircular ducts, and endolymphatic duct, and (2) a ventral saccular portion, which gives rise to the saccule and cochlear duct. The cochlear duct gives rise to the *spiral organ* (of Corti). The *bony labyrinth* develops from the mesenchyme adjacent to the membranous labyrinth (Fig. 14–9).

The epithelium lining the tympanic cavity, mastoid antrum, and auditory tube is derived from the endoderm of the *tubotympanic recess* that develops from the first pharyngeal pouch (Fig. 14–9, sketch 1). The auditory ossicles (malleus, incus, and stapes) develop from the dorsal ends of the cartilages of the first two branchial or pharyngeal arches (Fig. 14–9, sketch 2).

The epithelium of the *external acoustic meatus* develops from the ectoderm of the first branchial or pharyngeal groove (Fig. 14–9, sketch 1). The *tympanic membrane* is derived from three sources: (1) the endoderm of the first pharyngeal pouch, (2) the ectoderm of the first branchial or pharyngeal groove, and (3) the mesenchyme that grows between these layers (Fig. 14–9, sketch 3).

The auricle develops from six *auricular hillocks,* which result from mesenchymal swellings that develop around the margins of the first branchial or pharyngeal groove (Fig. 14–10). These hillocks fuse to form the definitive auricle.

Congenital deafness may result from abnormal development of the membranous labyrinth and/or bony labyrinth, as well as from abnormalities of the auditory ossicles. Recessive inheritance is the most common cause of congenital deafness, but a rubella virus infection near the end of the embryonic period is a major environmental factor known to cause abnormal development of the spiral organ and defective hearing.

There are many minor, clinically unimportant abnormalities of the auricle, but they alert the clinician to the possible presence of associated major anomalies (e.g., of the heart and kidneys). Low-set, severely malformed ears are often associated with chromosomal abnormalities, particularly trisomy 13 and trisomy 18 (see Chapter 5).

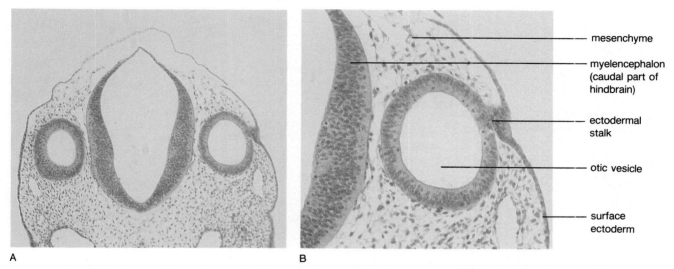

A   B

Figure 14-7. *A,* Photomicrograph of a transverse section of an embryo (×55) at Carnegie stage 12, about 26 days. (See Fig. 2-10 for the external appearance and size of an embryo at this stage). Observe the otic vesicles (auditory vesicles), the primordia of the membranous labyrinths, which give rise to the internal ears (Fig. 14-9). *B,* Higher magnification of the right otic vesicle (×120). Note the ectodermal stalk which is still attached to the remnant of the otic placode (Fig. 14-9*C*). (From Nishimura H (ed): *Atlas of Human Prenatal Histology.* Igaku-Shoin, Tokyo, 1983).

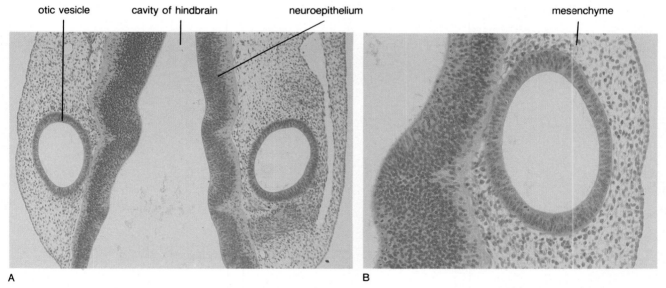

A   B

Figure 14-8. *A,* Photomicrograph of a transverse section of the embryo (×55), shown in Figure 14-7, at slightly more caudal level showing the otic vesicles lying free in the mesenchyme adjacent to the hindbrain. *B,* Higher magnification of the right otic vesicle (×120), the primordium of the membranous labyrinth (Fig. 14-9).

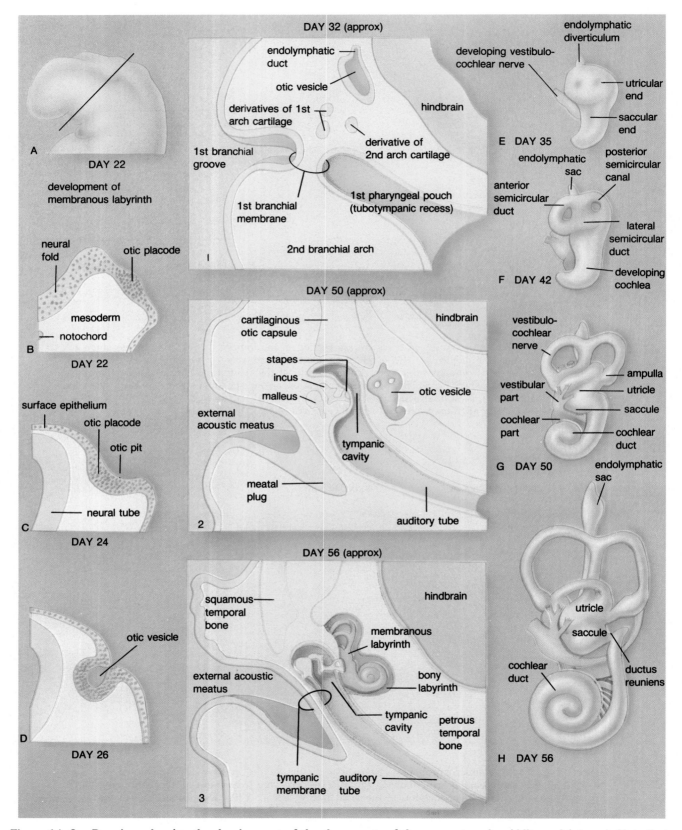

Figure 14-9. Drawings showing the development of the three parts of the ear; external, middle, and internal. Note that the otic placode (B), the first indication of the internal ear, appears first. The primordia of the middle and external parts of the ear appear about two days later.

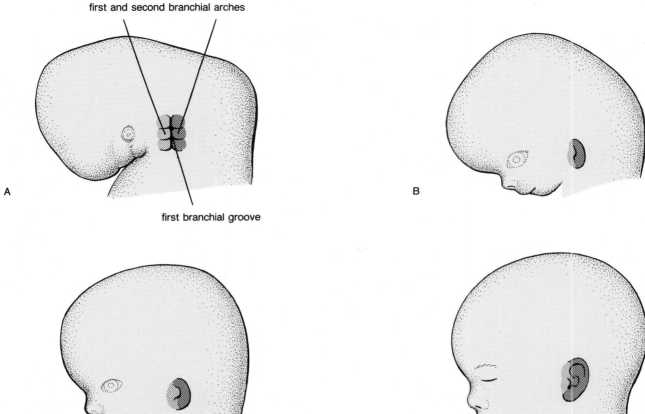

auricular hillocks derived from the
first and second branchial arches

A

first branchial groove

B

C

D

Figure 14–10. Drawings showing development of the auricle of the external ear. *A,* Six weeks. Note that three auricular hillocks are located on the first branchial or pharyngeal arch and three on the second arch. *B,* Eight weeks. The fused auricular hillocks are located on each side of the first branchial or pharyngeal groove, the primordium of the external acoustic (auditory) meatus. *C,* Ten weeks. *D,* Thirty-two weeks. As the jaws develop, the auricles move from the neck to the side of the head. (From Moore KL and Persaud TVN: *The Developing Human,* ed 5. Philadelphia, WB Saunders, 1993.)

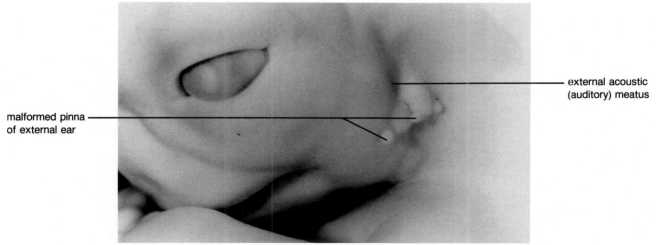

external acoustic
(auditory) meatus

malformed pinna
of external ear

Figure 14–11. Lateral view of the head and neck of an embryo at Carnegie stage 22, about 54 days, showing a severely malformed auricle (pinna). For the normal appearance of the auricle at this stage, see Figure 2–24. As fusion of the auricular hillocks to form the auricle is rather complicated, anomalies of the auricles (usually minor) are common. Minor deformities of the auricles may be clues to serious anomalies, e.g., of the kidneys. (From Nishimura H et al: *Prenatal Development of the Human with Special Reference to Craniofacial Structures: An Atlas.* U.S. Department of Health, Education, and Welfare, N.I.H., Bethesda, 1977.)

15

THE SKIN AND RELATED STRUCTURES

The skin and its appendages develop from ectoderm and mesoderm (Figs. 15–1 to 15–3). The **epidermis** is derived from ectoderm. The *melanocytes* are derived from *neural crest cells* that migrate into the epidermis. The **dermis** develops from mesenchyme that arises from mesoderm. Cast-off cells from the epidermis mix with secretions of the sebaceous glands to form a whitish, greasy coating for the skin known as *vernix caseosa.* It protects the epidermis, probably making it more waterproof, and facilitates birth due to its slipperiness.

Congenital anomalies of the skin are mainly *disorders of keratinization* (ichthyosis) and pigmentation (albinism). Abnormal blood vessel development results in various types of angioma.

HAIR

Hairs develop from downgrowths of the epidermis into the dermis (Fig. 15–2). By about 20 weeks the fetus is completely covered with fine, downy hairs called *lanugo.* These hairs are shed by birth or shortly thereafter and are replaced by coarser hairs.

GLANDS

Most *sebaceous glands* develop as outgrowths from the side of hair follicles (Fig. 15–2). Some sebaceous glands develop as downgrowths of the epidermis into the dermis. *Sweat glands* also develop from epidermal downgrowths into the dermis. *Mammary glands* develop in a similar manner (Fig. 15–3). Absence of mammary glands is rare, but supernumerary breasts (polymastia) or nipples (polythelia) are relatively common.

TEETH

Teeth develop from ectoderm and mesoderm. The enamel is produced by *ameloblasts,* which are derived from the oral ectoderm; all other dental tissues develop from neural crest-derived mesenchyme of the jaw.

TOOTH ERUPTION (FIGS. 15–4 AND 15–5).   As the teeth develop they begin a continuous movement externally. The mandibular teeth usually erupt before the maxillary teeth, and girls' teeth usually erupt sooner than boys' teeth. The child's dentition contains 20 deciduous teeth. The complete adult dentition consists of 32 teeth.

Text continued on page 236

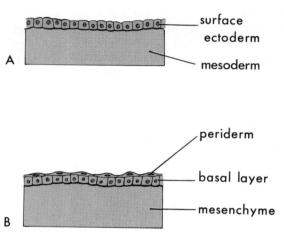

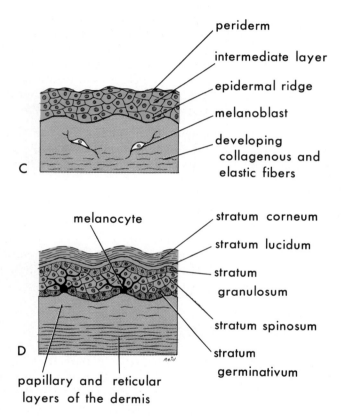

Figure 15-1. Drawings illustrating successive stages in the development of thick skin. The skin has a twofold origin: the epidermis develops from ectoderm and the dermis arises from mesoderm, the source of mesenchyme. *A,* Four weeks. *B,* Seven weeks. *C,* 11 weeks. The cells of the periderm continually undergo keratinization and desquamation. The exfoliated peridermal cells form part of the vernix caseosa, a white greasy substance that coats the fetal skin. *D,* Newborn. Note the position of the melanocytes in the basal layer of the epidermis and the way their branching processes extend between the epidermal cells to supply them with melanin. (From Moore KL and Persaud TVN: *The Developing Human,* ed 5. Philadelphia, WB Saunders, 1993.)

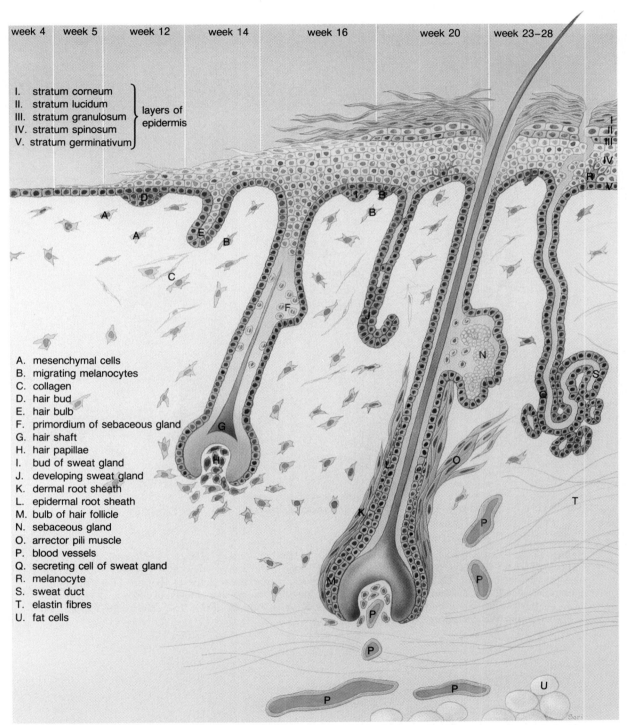

week 4   week 5   week 12   week 14   week 16   week 20   week 23–28

I.   stratum corneum
II. stratum lucidum   } layers of
III. stratum granulosum   } epidermis
IV. stratum spinosum
V.   stratum germinativum

A. mesenchymal cells
B. migrating melanocytes
C. collagen
D. hair bud
E. hair bulb
F. primordium of sebaceous gland
G. hair shaft
H. hair papillae
I. bud of sweat gland
J. developing sweat gland
K. dermal root sheath
L. epidermal root sheath
M. bulb of hair follicle
N. sebaceous gland
O. arrector pili muscle
P. blood vessels
Q. secreting cell of sweat gland
R. melanocyte
S. sweat duct
T. elastin fibres
U. fat cells

Figure 15–2.   Drawing illustrating development of the skin, a hair, and sebaceous and sweat glands.

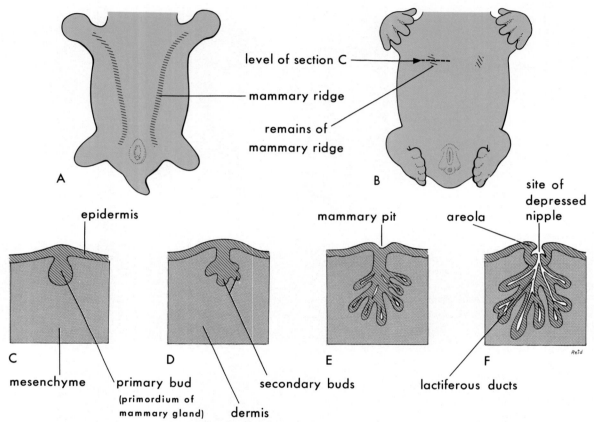

Figure 15–3. Drawings illustrating development of the mammary glands. *A,* Ventral view of an embryo of about 28 days, showing the mammary ridges. *B,* Similar view at six weeks showing the remains of these ridges. *C,* Transverse section through a mammary ridge at the site of a developing mammary gland. *D, E,* and *F,* Similar sections showing successive stages of breast development between the twelfth week and birth. (From Moore KL and Persaud TVN: *The Developing Human,* ed 5. Philadelphia, WB Saunders, 1993.)

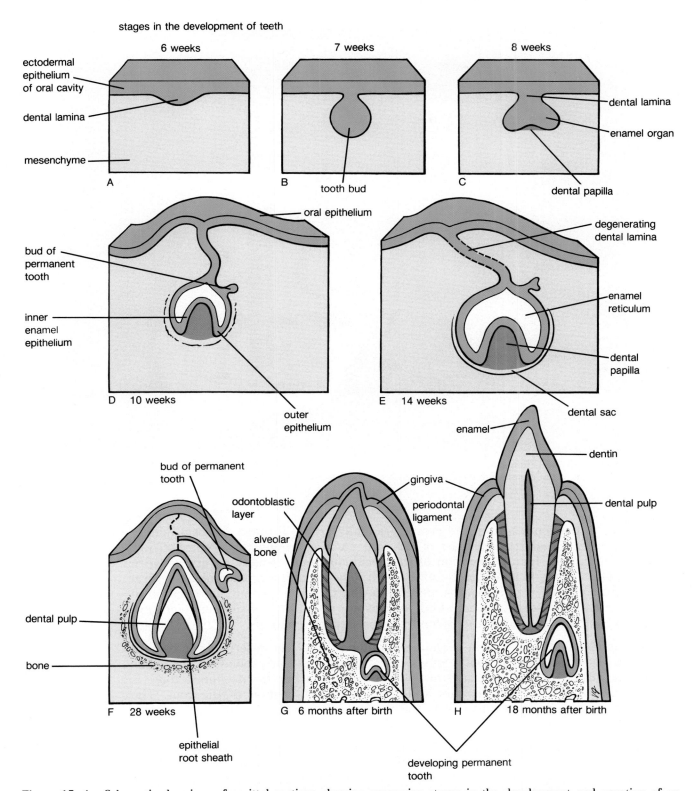

stages in the development of teeth

Figure 15-4. Schematic drawings of sagittal sections showing successive stages in the development and eruption of an incisor tooth. *A*, Six weeks, showing the dental lamina. *B*, Seven weeks, showing the tooth bud developing from the dental lamina. *C*, Eight weeks, showing the cap stage of tooth development. *D*, Ten weeks, showing the early bell stage of the deciduous tooth and the bud stage of the developing permanent tooth. *E*, Fourteen weeks, showing the advanced bell stage of the enamel organ. Note that the connection (dental lamina) of the tooth to the oral epithelium is degenerating. *F*, Twenty-eight weeks, showing the enamel and dentin layers. *G*, Six months postnatal showing early tooth eruption. *H*, Eighteen months postnatal, showing a fully erupted deciduous incisor tooth. The permanent incisor tooth now has a well-developed crown.

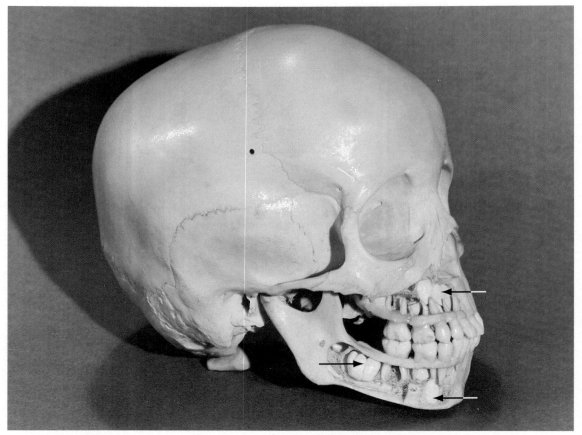

Figure 15-5. Photograph of a four-year-old child's skull. The bone has been removed to show the relations of the developing permanent teeth *(arrows)* to the erupted deciduous teeth.

As the root of the tooth grows, the crown gradually erupts through the oral epithelium (Fig. 15–4*G* and *H*). The part of the oral mucosa around the erupted crown becomes the *gingiva* (gum). Eruption of the deciduous teeth usually occurs between the sixth and twenty-fourth months after birth. The mandibular medial or central incisors usually erupt 6 to 8 months after birth, but this process may not begin until 12 or 13 months in some normal children. Despite this, all 20 deciduous teeth are usually present by the end of the second year in healthy children.

The permanent teeth develop in a manner similar to that just described for deciduous teeth. As a permanent tooth grows, the root of the corresponding deciduous tooth is gradually resorbed by osteoclasts. Consequently, when the deciduous tooth is shed, it consists of the crown only and the uppermost portion of the root. The permanent teeth usually begin to erupt during the sixth year and continue to appear until early adulthood.

The common congenital anomalies of teeth are defective formation of enamel and dentin, abnormalities in shape, and variations in number and position. All tetracyclines are extensively incorporated into the enamel of developing teeth and produce brownish-yellow discoloration and hypoplasia of the enamel. Consequently, they are not administered during pregnancy and to children.

REFERENCES AND SUGGESTED READING

CHAPTER 1

Alpin JD: Implantation, trophoblast differentiation and hemochorial placentation: mechanistic evidence *in vivo* and *in vitro*. *J Cell Sci 99:*681, 1991.

Ash KM, Lyons ES, Levi CS, Lindsay DJ: Endovaginal sonographic diagnosis of ectopic twin gestation. *J Ultrasound Med 10:*497, 1991.

Edwards RG: A decade of *in vitro* fertilization. *Research in Reprod 22:*1, 1990.

Filly RA: Ectopic pregnancy. *In* Callen PW (ed): *Ultrasonography in Obstetrics and Gynecology,* 2nd ed. Philadelphia, WB Saunders, 1988.

Fugger EP, Bustillo M, Dorfmann AD, Schulman JD: Human preimplantation embryo cryopreservation: selected aspects. *Human Reprod 6:*131, 1991.

Moore KL, Persaud TVN: *The Developing Human: Clinically Oriented Embryology,* 5th ed. Philadelphia, WB Saunders, 1993.

Nahhas F, Barnea E: Human embryonic origin of early pregnancy factor before and after implantation. *Am J Reprod Immunol 22:*105, 1990.

O'Rahilly R, Müller F: *Developmental Stages in Human Embryos.* Washington, Carnegie Institute of Washington, 1987.

O'Rahilly R, Müller F: *Human Embryology & Teratology.* New York, Wiley-Liss, 1992.

Steinkampf MP, Kretzer PA, McElroy E, Conway-Myers BA: A simplified approach to in vitro fertilization. *J Reprod Med 37:*199, 1992.

Wood C, Trouson A (eds): *Clinical In Vitro Fertilization,* 2nd ed. New York, Springer Verlag, 1989.

CHAPTER 2

Barnea ER, Hustin J, Jauniaux E (eds): *The First Twelve Weeks of Gestation.* Berlin, Springer-Verlag, 1992.

Biggers JD: Arbitrary Partitions of Prenatal Life. *Human Reprod 5:*1, 1990.

Chapman MG, Grudzinskas JG, Chard T (eds): *The Embryo: Normal and Abnormal Development and Growth.* New York, Springer-Verlag, 1990.

Filly RA: The first trimester. *In* Callen PW (ed): *Ultrasonography in Obstetrics and Gynecology,* 2nd ed. Philadelphia, WB Saunders, 1988.

Gasser RF: *Atlas of Human Embryos.* Hagerstown, Harper & Row, 1975.

Holzgreve W, Flake AW, Langer JC: The fetus with sacrococcygeal teratoma. *In* Harrison MR, Golbus MS, Filly RA (eds): *The Unborn Patient: Prenatal Diagnosis and Treatment,* 2nd ed. Philadelphia, WB Saunders, 1991.

Kalousek DK, Fitch N, Paradice BA: *Pathology of the Human Embryo and Previable Fetus: An Atlas.* New York, Springer-Verlag, 1990.

Navaratnam V: Organization and reorganization of blood vessels in embryonic development. *Eye 5(Pt.2):*147, 1991.

Nishimura H (ed): *Atlas of Human Prenatal Histology.* Tokyo, Igaku-Shoin, 1983.

Nishimura H, Semba R, Tanimura T, Uwabe C: Normal development of early human embryos: Observation of 90 specimens at Carnegie stages 7 to 13. *Teratology 10:*1, 1974.

O'Rahilly R, Müller F: *Developmental Stages in Human Embryos.* Washington, Carnegie Institute of Washington, 1987.

O'Rahilly R, Müller F: Human Embryology & Teratology. New York, Wiley-Liss, 1992.

Schats R, Van Os HC, Jansen CAM, Wladimiroff JW: The crown-rump length in early human pregnancy: a reappraisal. *Br J Obstet Gynaecol 98:*460, 1991.

Shiota K: Development and intrauterine fate of normal and abnormal human conceptuses. *Cong Anom 31:*67, 1991.

Smith JL, Schoenwolf GC: Further evidence of extrinsic forces in bending of the neural plate. *J Comp Neurol 307:*225, 1991.

CHAPTER 3

Birnholz JC, Benaceraff BR: The development of human fetal hearing. *Science 222*:516, 1983.

Boehm CD, Kazazian Jr, HH: Prenatal diagnosis by DNA analysis. *In* Harrison MR, Golbus MS, Filly RA (eds): *The Unborn Patient: Prenatal Diagnosis and Treatment,* 2nd ed. Philadelphia, WB Saunders, 1991.

Bowie JD: Fetal growth. *In* Callen PW (ed): *Ultrasonography in Obstetrics and Gynecology,* 2nd ed. Philadelphia, WB Saunders, 1988.

England MA: *Color Atlas of Life Before Birth.* Chicago, Year Book Medical Publishers, 1983.

Filly RA: Sonographic anatomy of the normal fetus. *In* Harrison MR, Golbus MS, Filly RA (eds): *The Unborn Patient: Prenatal Diagnosis and Treatment,* 2nd ed. Philadelphia, WB Saunders, 1991.

Haddow JE: α-Fetoprotein. *In* Harrison MR, Golbus MS, Filly RA (eds): *The Unborn Patient: Prenatal Diagnosis and Treatment,* 2nd ed. Philadelphia, WB Saunders, 1991.

Harrison MR: Selection for treatment: Which defects are correctable. *In* Harrison MR, Golbus MS, Filly RA (eds): *The Unborn Patient: Prenatal Diagnosis and Treatment,* 2nd ed. Philadelphia, WB Saunders, 1991.

Hobbins JC: Amniocentesis. *In* Harrison MR, Golbus MS, Filly RA (eds): *The Unborn Patient: Prenatal Diagnosis and Treatment,* 2nd ed. Philadelphia, WB Saunders, 1991.

Hogge WA: Chorionic villus sampling. *In* Harrison MR, Golbus, MS, Filly RA (eds): *The Unborn Patient: Prenatal Diagnosis and Treatment,* 2nd ed. Philadelphia, WB Saunders, 1991.

Kurtz AB, Needleman L: Ultrasound assessment of fetal age. *In* Callen PW (ed): *Ultrasonography in Obstetrics and Gynecology.* Philadelphia, WB Saunders, 1988.

Simpson JL, Elias S: Prenatal diagnosis of genetic disorders. *In* Creasy RK, Resnik R (eds): *Maternal-Fetal Medicine: Principals and Practice,* 2nd ed. Philadelphia, WB Saunders, 1989.

Thompson MW, McInnes RR, Willard HF: *Thompson & Thompson: Genetics in Medicine,* 5th ed. Philadelphia, WB Saunders, 1991.

Wald NJ, Cuckle HS: AFP screening in early pregnancy. *In* Spencer JAD (ed): *Fetal Monitoring.* Oxford, Oxford University Press, 1991.

CHAPTER 4

Bassett JM: Current perspectives on placental development and its integration with fetal growth. *Proc Nutr Soc 50*:311, 1991.

Bernischke K, Kaufman P: *The Pathology of the Human Placenta.* Berlin, Springer-Verlag, 1990.

Filly RA: The first trimester. *In* Callen PW (ed): *Ultrasonography in Obstetrics and Gynecology,* 2nd ed. Philadelphia, WB Saunders, 1988.

Hay WW: In vivo measurements of placental transport and metabolism. *Proc Nutr Soc 50*:355, 1991.

Jauniaux E, Campbell S: Ultrasonographic assessment of placental abnormalities. *Am J Obstet Gynecol 163*:1650, 1990.

Lindsay DJ, Lovett IS, Lyons EA, Levi CS, Zheng X-H, Holt SC, Daschefsky SM: Endovaginal sonography: Yolk sac diameter and shape as a predictor of pregnancy outcome in the first trimester. *Radiology 183*:115, 1992.

Lyons EA, Levi CS: Ultrasound of the normal first trimester of pregnancy. Syllabus. Special Course. Ultrasound, Radiological Society of North America, 1991.

Moore KL, Persaud TVN: *The Developing Human: Clinically Oriented Embryology,* 5th ed. Philadelphia, WB Saunders, 1993.

Naeye RL: *Disorders of the Placenta, Fetus, and Neonate.* St. Louis, Mosby-year Book, 1992.

Nyberg DA, Callen PW: Ultrasound evaluation of the placenta. *In* Callen PW (ed): *Ultrasonography in Obstetrics and Gynecology,* 2nd ed. Philadelphia, WB Saunders, 1988.

Peipert JF, Donnenfeld AE, Oligohydramnios: A review. *Obstet Gynecol 46*:325, 1991.

Petraglia F, Angioni S, Coukos G, Uccelli E, Didomenica P, Deramundo BM, Genazzani Ad, Garuti GC, Segre A: Neuroendocrine mechanisms regulating placental hormone production. *Contr Gynecol Obstet 18*:147, 1991.

Schneider H: Placental transport function. *Reprod Fert Develop 3*:345, 1991.

CHAPTER 5

Briggs GG, Freeman RK, Yaffe SJ: *Drugs in Pregnancy and Lactation,* 3rd ed. Baltimore, Williams & Wilkins, 1990.

Buitendijk S, Bracken MB: Medication in early pregnancy: Prevalence of use and relationship to maternal characteristics. *Am J Obstet Gynecol 165*:33, 1991.

Burbacher TM, Rodier PM, Weiss B: Methylmercury developmental neurotoxicity: A comparison of effects in humans and animals. *Neurotoxicol Teratol 12*:191, 1990.

Dansky LV, Finnell RH: Parental epilepsy, anticonvulsant drugs, and reproductive outcome: Epidemiologic and experimental findings spanning 3 decades. 2. Human studies. *Reprod Toxicol 5*:301, 1991.

Day N, Sambamoorthi V, Taylor P, Richardson G, Robles N, Jhon Y, Scher M, Stoffer D, Cornelius M, Jasperse D: Prenatal marijuana use and neonatal outcome. *Neurotoxicol Teratol 13*:329, 1991.

Dimmick JE, Kalousek DK (eds): *Developmental Pathology of the Embryo and Fetus.* Philadelphia, JB Lippincott, 1992.

Fantel AG, Shephard TH: Prenatal cocaine exposure. *Reprod Toxicol 4*:83, 1990.

Ginsburg KA, Blacker CM, Abel EL, Sokol RJ: Fetal alcohol exposure and adverse pregnancy outcome. *Contr Gynecol Obstet 18*:115, 1991.

Graham JM Jr: *Smith's Recognizable Patterns of Human Deformation,* 2nd ed. Philadelphia, WB Saunders, 1988.

Greenough A, Osborne J, Sutherland S (eds): *Congenital, Perinatal and Neonatal Infections.* Edinburgh, Churchill Livingstone, 1992.

Hanssens M, Keirse MJNC, Vankelecom F, Van Assche FA: Fetal and neonatal effects of treatment with angiotensin-converting enzyme inhibitors in pregnancy. *Obstet Gynecol 78*:128, 1991.

Holmes LB: Teratogens. *In* Behrman RE (ed): *Nelson Textbook of Pediatrics,* 14th ed. Philadelphia, WB Saunders, 1992.

Jones KL: *Smith's Recognizable Patterns of Human Malformation,* 4th ed. Philadelphia, WB Saunders, 1988.

Koren G (ed): *Maternal-Fetal Toxicology: A Clinician's Guide.* New York, Marcel Dekker, 1990.

Laegreid L, Olegard R, Walstrom J, Conradi N: Teratogenic effects of benzodiazepine use during pregnancy. *J Pediatr 114*:126, 1989.

Moore KL, Persaud TVN: *The Developing Human: Clinically Oriented Embryology,* 5th ed. Philadelphia, WB Saunders, 1993.

Nishimura H, Okamoto N: *Sequential Atlas of Human Congenital Malformations. Observations of Embryos, Fetuses and Newborns.* Tokyo, Igaku-Shoin, 1976.

Nishimura H, Tanimura T: *Clinical Aspects of the Teratogenicity of Drugs.* Amsterdam, Excerpta Medica/New York, American Elsevier, 1976.

Persaud TVN: *Environmental Causes of Human Birth Defects.* Springfield, Charles C Thomas, 1990.

Persaud TVN, Chudley AE, Skalko RG: *Basic Concepts in Teratology.* New York, Alan R. Liss, 1985.

Remington JS, Klein JO (eds): *Infectious Diseases of the Fetus and Newborn Infant,* 3rd ed. Philadelphia, WB Saunders, 1990.

Shepard TH: *Catalog of Teratogenic Agents,* 7th ed. Baltimore, The Johns Hopkins University Press, 1992.

Shepard TH, Fantel AG, Fitzsimmons J: Congenital defect rates among spontaneous abortuses: Twenty years of monitoring. *Teratology 39*:325, 1989.

Thompson MW, McInnes RR, Willard HF: *Thompson & Thompson: Genetics in Medicine,* 5th ed. Philadelphia, WB Saunders, 1991.

CHAPTER 6

Goldstein RB, Callen PW: Ultrasound evaluation of the fetal thorax and abdomen. *In* Callen PW: *Ultrasonography in Obstetrics and Gynecology,* 2nd ed. Philadelphia, WB Saunders, 1988.

Harrison MR: The fetus with a diaphragmatic hernia: Pathophysiology, natural history, and surgical management. *In* Harrison MR, Golbus MS, Filly RA (eds): *The Unborn Patient: Prenatal Diagnosis and Treatment,* 2nd ed. Philadelphia, WB Saunders, 1991.

McNamara JJ, Eraklis AJ, Gross RE: Congenital posterolateral diaphragmatic hernia in the newborn. *J Thorac Cardiovasc Surg 55*:55, 1968.

Moore KL, Persaud TVN: *The Developing Human: Clinically Oriented Embryology,* 5th ed. Philadelphia, WB Saunders, 1991.

Reynolds M: Diaphragmatic anomalies. *In* Raffensperger JG (ed): *Swenson's Pediatric Surgery,* 5th ed. Norwalk, Appleton & Lange, 1990.

Taeusch HW, Ballard RA, Avery ME (eds): *Schaffer and Avery's Diseases of the Newborn,* 6th ed. Philadelphia, WB Saunders, 1991.

CHAPTER 7

Chetty R, Forder MD: Parathyroiditis associated with hyperthyroidism and branchial cysts. *Am J Clin Path 96*:348, 1991.

Ferguson MWJ: Palate development. *Development 103(Suppl)*:41, 1988.

Gorlin RJ, Cohen Jr, MM, Levin LS: *Syndromes of the Head and Neck,* 3rd ed. New York, Oxford Univ Press, 1990.

Greene RM: Signal transduction during craniofacial development. *Critical Rev Toxicol 20*:153, 1989.

Hall BK: Mechanisms of craniofacial development. *In* Vig KWL, Burdi AR (eds): *Craniofacial Morphogenesis and Dysmorphogenesis.* Ann Arbor, The University of Michigan, 1988.

Hinrichsen K: *The Early Development of Morphology and Patterns of the Face in the Human Embryo. Advances in Anatomy, Embryology and Cell Biology 98.* New York, Springer-Verlag, 1985.

Jones KL: Smith's *Recognizable Patterns of Human Malformation,* 4th ed. Philadelphia, WB Saunders, 1988.

Kendall MD: Functional anatomy of the thymic microenvironment. *J Anat 177:*1, 1991.

Miyauchi A, Matsuzuka F, Kuma K, Katayama S: Piriform sinus fistula and the ultimobranchial body. *Histopath 20:*221, 1992.

Moore KL, Persaud TVN: *The Developing Human: Clinically Oriented Embryology,* 5th ed. Philadelphia, WB Saunders, 1993.

Niermeyer MF, Van der Meulen JC: Genetics of craniofacial malformations. *In* Stricker M, Van der Meulen JC, Raphael B, Mazzola R (eds): *Craniofacial Malformations.* Edinburgh, Churchill Livingstone, 1990.

Nishimura H, Semba R, Tanimura T, Tanaka O: *Prenatal Development of the Human with Special Reference to Craniofacial Structures: An Atlas.* US Department of Health, Education, and Welfare, National Institutes of Health, Bethesda, 1977.

Pfeifer G (ed): *Craniofacial Abnormalities and Clefts of the Lip, Alveolus and Palate.* New York, Georg Thieme Verlag, 1991.

Schubert J, Schmidt R, Raupach H-W: New findings explaining the mode of action in prevention of facial clefting and first clinical experience. *J Cranio-Max Fac Surg 18:*343, 1990.

Sperber GH: *Craniofacial Embryology,* 4th ed. London, Butterworth, 1989.

Stricker M, Raphael B, Van der Meulen J, Mazzola R: Craniofacial growth and development. *In* Stricker M, Van der Meulen JC, Raphael B, Mazzola R (eds): *Craniofacial Malformations.* Edinburgh, Churchill Livingstone, 1990.

van der Meulen J, Mozzola B, Stricker M, Raphael B: Classification of craniofacial malformations. *In* Stricker M, Van der Meulen JC, Raphael B, Mazzola R (eds): *Craniofacial Malformations.* Edinburgh, Churchill Livingstone, 1990.

Vermeij-Keers C: Craniofacial embryology and morphogenesis: normal and abnormal. *In* Stricker M, Van der Meulen JC, Raphael B, Mazzola R (eds): *Craniofacial Malformations.* Edinburgh, Churchill Livingstone, 1990.

CHAPTER 8

Ballard PL: Hormonal control of lung maturation. *Bailliere's Clin Endocrin Metabol 3:*723, 1989.

Chernick V, Kryger MH: Pediatric lung disease. *In* Kryger MH (ed): *Introduction to Respiratory Medicine,* 2nd ed. New York, Churchill Livingstone, 1990.

De Vries PA, De Vries CR: Embryology and development. *In* Othersen Jr, HB (ed): *The Pediatric Airway.* Philadelphia, WB Saunders, 1991.

Harrison MR: The fetus with a diaphragmatic hernia: Pathology, natural history, and surgical management. *In* Harrison MR, Golbus MS, Filly RA: *The Unborn Patient: Prenatal Diagnosis and Treatment,* 2nd ed. Philadelphia, WB Saunders, 1991.

Kozuma S, Nemoto A, Okai T, Mizuno M: Maturational sequence of fetal breathing movements. *Biol Neonate 60(suppl 1):*36, 1991.

Moore KL, Persaud TVN: *The Developing Human: Clinically Oriented Embryology,* 5th ed. Philadelphia, WB Saunders, 1993.

Patrick J, Gagnon R: Fetal breathing and body movement. *In* Creasy RK, Resnik R (eds): *Maternal-Fetal Medicine: Principles and Practice,* 2nd ed. Philadelphia, WB Saunders, 1989.

Scarpelli EM (ed): *Pulmonary Physiology: Fetus, Newborn, Child and Adolescent,* 2nd ed. Philadelphia, Lea and Febiger, 1990.

Whitsett JA: Molecular aspects of the pulmonary surfactant system in the newborn. *In* Chernick V, Mellins RB (eds): *Basic Mechanisms of Pediatric Respiratory Disease: Cellular and Integrative.* Philadelphia, BC Decker, 1991.

CHAPTER 9

Beasley SW, Myers NA, Auldist AW (eds): *Oesophageal Atresia.* London, Chapman and Hall, 1991.

Best LG, Wiseman NE, Chudley AE: Familial duodenal atresia: a report of two families and review. *Am J Med Genet 34:*442, 1989.

Brassett C, Ellis H: Transposition of the viscera. *Clin Anat 4:*139, 1991.

Cobb RA, Williamson RCN: Embryology and developmental abnormalities of the large intestine. *In* Phillips SF, Pemberton JH, Shorter RG (eds): *The Large Intestine: Physiology, Pathophysiology, and Disease.* New York, Raven Press, 1991.

Filly RA: Sonographic anatomy of the normal fetus. *In* Harrison MR, Golbus MS, Filly RA (eds): *The Unborn Patient: Prenatal Diagnosis and Treatment,* 2nd ed. Philadelphia, WB Saunders, 1991.

Herbst JJ: Disorders of the esophagus. *In* Behrman RE (ed): *Nelson Textbook of Pediatrics,* 14th ed. Philadelphia, WB Saunders, 1992.

Kleigman RM, Behrman RE: The umbilicus. *In* Behrman RE (ed): *Nelson Textbook of Pediatrics,* 14th ed. Philadelphia, WB Saunders, 1992.

Moore KL, Persaud TVN: *The Developing Human: Clinically Oriented Embryology*, 5th ed. Philadelphia, WB Saunders, 1993.

Noordijk JA: Omphalocele and gastroschisis. *In* Persaud TVN (ed): *Advances in the Study of Birth Defects, vol. 6. Cardiovascular, Respiratory, Gastrointestinal and Genitourinary Malformations.* New York, Alan R Liss, 1982.

Shandling B: Congenital and perinatal anomalies of the gastrointestinal tract and intestinal rotation. *In* Behrman RE (ed): *Nelson Textbook of Pediatrics*, 14th ed. Philadelphia, WB Saunders, 1992.

Thompson JC: *Atlas of Surgery of the Stomach, Duodenum, and Small Bowel.* St. Louis, Mosby Year Book, 1992.

CHAPTER 10

DiGeorge AM: Hermaphroditism. *In* Behrman RE (ed): *Nelson Textbook of Pediatrics*, 14th ed. Philadelphia, WB Saunders, 1992.

Mittwoch U: Sex determination and sex reversal: genotype, phenotype, dogma and semantics. *Human Genet 89*:467, 1992.

Moore KL and Persaud TVN: *The Developing Human: Clinically Oriented Embryology*, 5th ed. Philadelphia, WB Saunders, 1993.

Persaud TVN: Embryology of the female genital tract and gonads. *In* Copeland LJ, Jarrell J, McGregor J (eds): *Textbook of Gynecology.* Philadelphia, WB Saunders, 1993.

Rutgers JL: Advances in the pathology of intersex conditions. *Hum Path 22*:884, 1991.

Thompson MW, McInnes RR, Willard HF: *Thompson & Thompson: Genetics in Medicine*, 5th ed. Philadelphia, WB Saunders, 1991.

CHAPTER 11

Chinn A, Fitzsimmons J, Shepard TH, Fantel AG: Congenital heart disease among spontaneous abortuses and stillborn fetuses: Prevalence and associations. *Teratology 40*:475, 1989.

Deanfield JE: Transposition of the great arteries: To switch or not to switch? *Curr Opin Pediatr 1*:85, 1989.

Feinberg RN, Sherer GK, Auerbach R (eds): *The Development of the Vascular System.* Basel, Karger, 1991.

Kirklin JW, Colvin EV, McConnell ME, et al.: Complete transposition of the great arteries: Treatment in the current era. *Pediatr Clin North Am 37*:171, 1990.

Long WA: *Fetal and Neonatal Cardiology.* Philadelphia, WB Saunders, 1990.

Moore KL, Persaud TVN: *The Developing Human: Clinically Oriented Embryology*, 5th ed. Philadelphia, WB Saunders, 1993.

Schats R, Jansen CAM, Wladimiroff JW: Embryonic heart activity: Appearance and development in early pregnancy. *Brit J Obstet Gynaecol 97*:989, 1990.

Schmidt KG, Silverman WH: The fetus with a cardiac malformation. *In* Harrison MR, Golbus MS, Filly RA (eds): *The Unborn Patient: Prenatal Diagnosis and Treatment*, 2nd ed. Philadelphia, WB Saunders, 1991.

Skovránek J: Prenatal development of the heart and the blood circulatory system. *Physiol Res 40*:25, 1991.

Ueland K: Cardiac diseases. *In* Creasy RK, Resnik R (eds): *Maternal-Fetal Medicine: Principles and Practice.* Philadelphia, WB Saunders, 1989.

Virmani R, Atkinson JD, Fenoglio JJ: *Cardiovascular Pathology.* Philadelphia, WB Saunders, 1991.

CHAPTER 12

Bruder SP, Caplan AL: Cellular and molecular events during embryonic bone development. *Connect Tissue Res 20*:65, 1989.

Cole DEC, Cohen Jr, MM: Osteogenesis imperfecta: An update. *J Pediatr 119*:73, 1991.

Cormack DH: *Essential Histology.* Philadelphia, WB Saunders, 1993.

Daniels K, Solursh M: Modulation of chondrogenesis by the cytoskeleton and extracellular matrix. *J Cell Sci 100 (Pt. 2)*:249, 1991.

Dziedzic-Goclawska A, Emerich J, Grzesik W, Stachowicz W, Michalik J, Ostrowski K: Differences in the kinetics of the mineralization process in endochondral and intramembranous osteogenesis in human fetal development. *J Bone Miner Res 3*:533, 1988.

Marin-Padilla M: Cephalic axial skeletal-neural dysraphic disorders: Embryology and pathology. *Can J Neurol Sci 18*:153, 1991.

Moore KL, Persaud TVN: *The Developing Human: Clinically Oriented Embryology*, 5th ed. Philadelphia, WB Saunders, 1993.

O'Rahilly R, Müller F, Meyer DB: The human vertebral column at the end of the embryonic period proper. 3. The thoracolumbar region. *J Anat 168*:81, 1990a.

O'Rahilly R, Müller F, Meyer DB: The human vertebral column at the end of the embryonic period proper. 4. The sacrococcygeal region. *J Anat 168:*95, 1990b.

Stedman H, Sarkar S: Molecular genetics in basic myology: A rapidly evolving perspective. *Muscle Nerve II:*668, 1988.

Uhthoff HK: *The Embryology of the Human Locomotor System.* New York, Springer-Verlag, 1990.

Van Allen MI: Structural anomalies resulting from vascular disruption. *Pediatr Clin NA 39:*255, 1992.

van der Harten HJ, Brons JT, Schipper NW, Dijkstra PF, Meijer CJ, van Geijin HP: The prenatal development of the normal human skeleton: a combined ultrasonographic and post-mortem radiographic study. *Pediatr Radiol 21:*52, 1990.

CHAPTER 13

Adams J: Prenatal exposure to teratogenic agents and neurodevelopmental outcome. *Research in Infant Assessment (BD:OAS)25:*63, 1989.

Alvarez IS, Schoenwolf GC: Expansion of surface epithelium provides the major extrinsic force for bending of the neural plate. *J Exp Zool 26:*340, 1992.

Cockroft DL: Vitamin deficiency and neural tube defects: human and animal studies. *Hum Reprod 6:*148, 1991.

Flint G: Embryology of the nervous system. *Br J Neurosurg 3:*131, 1989.

Greenough A, Osborne J, Sutherland S (eds): *Congenital, Perinatal and Neonatal Infections.* Edinburgh Churchill Livingstone, 1992.

Jacobson M: *Developmental Neurobiology,* 3rd ed. New York, Plenum Publishing, 1992.

Moore KL, Persaud TVN: *The Developing Human: Clinically Oriented Embryology,* 5th ed. Philadelphia, WB Saunders, 1993.

Müller F, O'Rahilly R: The development of the human brain from a closed neural tube at stage 13. *Anat Embryol (Berl) 177:*55, 1988.

Müller F, O'Rahilly R: Development of anencephaly and its variants. *Am J Anat 190:*193, 1991.

Persaud TVN: Abnormal development of the central nervous system. *Anat Anz 150:*44, 1981.

Persaud TVN: *Environmental Causes of Human Birth Defects.* Springfield, Charles C Thomas, 1990.

Sanes JR: Extracellular matrix molecules that influence neural development. *Annu Rev Neurosci 12:*491, 1989.

Schoenwolf GG, Smith JL: Mechanisms of neurulation: traditional viewpoint and recent advances. *Development 109:*243, 1990.

CHAPTER 14

Ars B: Organogenesis of the middle ear structures. *J Laryngol Otol 103:*16, 1989.

Birnholz JC: The development of human fetal eye movement patterns. *Science 213:*679, 1981.

Birnholz JC, Benaceraff BR: The development of human fetal hearing. *Science 222:*516, 1983.

Martyn LJ: Pediatric ophthalmology. *In* Behrman RE (ed): *Textbook of Pediatrics,* 14th ed. Philadelphia, WB Saunders, 1992.

Michaels L: Evolution of the epidermoid formation and its role in the development of the middle ear and tympanic membrane during the first trimester. *J Otolaryngol 17:*22, 1988.

Moll M: Congenital earpits or auricular sinuses. *Acta Path Microbiol Scand 99:*96, 1991.

Moore KL, Persaud TVN: *The Developing Human: Clinically Oriented Embryology,* 5th ed. Philadelphia, WB Saunders 1993.

Parrish KL, Amedee RG: Atresia of the external auditory canal. *J La State Med Soc 142:*9, 1990.

Sevel D, Isaacs R: A re-evaluation of corneal development. *Trans Am Ophthalmol Soc 86:*178, 1989.

Shah CP, Halperin DS: Congenital deafness. *In* Persaud TVN (ed): *Advances in the Study of Birth Defects, vol 7. Central Nervous System and Craniofacial Malformations.* New York, Alan R Liss, 1982.

Stromland K, Miller M, Cook C: Ocular teratology. *Surv Ophthalmol 35:*429, 1991.

Tripathi BJ, Tripathi RC, Livingston AM, Borisuth NSC: The role of growth factors in the embryogenesis and differentiation of the eye. *Am J Anat 192:*442, 1991.

CHAPTER 15

Beller F: Development and anatomy of the breast. *In* Mitchell Jr, GW, Bassett LW (eds): *The Female Breast and Its Disorders.* Baltimore, Williams & Wilkins, 1990.

Bland KI, Copeland III, EM (eds): *The Breast.* Philadelphia, WB Saunders, 1991.

Booth DH, Persaud TVN: Congenital absence of the breast. *Anat Anz 155:*23, 1984.

Haagensen CD: *Diseases of the Breast,* 3rd ed. Philadelphia, WB Saunders, 1986.

Hirschhorn K: Dermatoglyphics. *In* Behrman RE (ed): *Nelson Textbook of Pediatrics,* 14th ed. Philadelphia, WB Saunders, 1992.

Horn TD: Developmental defects of the skin. *In* Farmer ER, Hood AF (eds): *Pathology of the Skin.* Norwalk, Appleton & Lange, 1990.

Moore KL, Persaud TVN: *The Developing Human: Clinically Oriented Embryology,* 5th ed. Philadelphia, W.B. Saunders, 1993.

Müller M, Jasmin JR, Monteil RA, Loubiere R: Embryology of the hair follicle. *Early Hum Dev 26:*159, 1991.

Osborne MP: Breast development and anatomy. *In* Harris JR, Hellman S, Henderson IC, Kinne DW (eds): *Breast Diseases,* 2nd ed. Philadelphia, JB Lippincott, 1991.

Persaud TVN: *Environmental Causes of Human Birth Defects.* Springfield, Charles C Thomas, 1990.

Sperber GH: *Craniofacial Embryology,* 4th ed. London, Butterworth, 1989.

Ten Cate AR: Development of the tooth. *In* Ten Cate AR (ed): *Oral Histology: Structure and Function.* St. Louis, CV Mosby, 1989.

INDEX